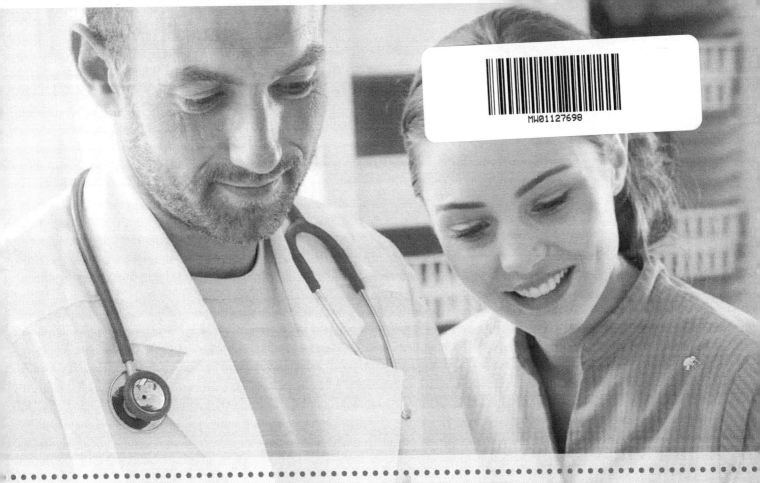

GR🟋ACE
PRESCRIPTIONS

BY WALT LARIMORE, MD & WILLIAM C. PEEL, THM

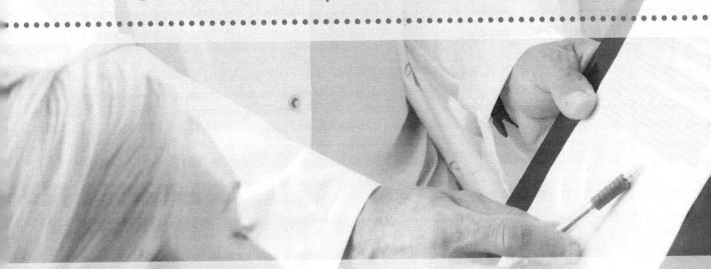

LEARNING TO SHARE YOUR FAITH IN YOUR PRACTICE

The Christian Medical & Dental Associations was founded in 1931 and currently serves more than 16,000 members; coordinates a network of Christian healthcare professionals for personal and professional growth; sponsors student ministries in medical and dental schools; conducts overseas healthcare projects for underserved populations; addresses policies on healthcare, medical ethics and bioethical and human rights issues; distributes educational and inspirational resources; provides missionary healthcare professionals with continuing education resources; and conducts international academic exchange programs.

For more information:
Christian Medical & Dental Associations
P.O. Box 7500
Bristol, TN 37621-7500
888-230-2637
www.cmda.org • main@cmda.org

ISBN 978-0-9706631-5-3
2013944822

Printed in the United States of America

In Memory of
Wayne Sanders
who, like Andrew, was always bringing
people to meet his Savior.

Wayne was responsible for linking Walt and Bill, and
he made *The Saline Solution* possible by hosting the
first live conference to see if anyone would come.

To Gene Rudd, MD

Through his tireless efforts, ...

astonishing humility as a man,
persistent vision as a leader,
exemplary practice as a grace-prescribing physician,
and extraordinary commitment as a friend,

... *Grace Prescriptions* became a reality.

TABLE OF CONTENTS

FOREWORD
by David Stevens, MD, MA (Ethics)

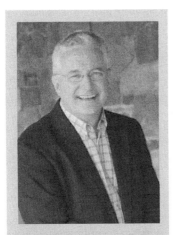

Dr. David Stevens is the CEO of Christian Medical & Dental Associations.

Witnessing to Christ's work in your life is not an option; it's an imperative. Christ's final command before He ascended into heaven was that His disciples be witnesses (Acts 1:8). Pointing people to Christ is a mandate, but also an incredible opportunity. Those of us who serve in the medical and dental professions have the best opportunities to point individuals toward Christ.

Most people will never enter a church, turn on a Christian radio station, or pick up a religious magazine, but everyone will eventually get sick. When they do, they will be thinking about their mortality, their lifestyle, and where they will spend eternity. If our patients are seriously ill, they may be praying for the first time in years. They trust their doctors with their most intimate details. They seek advice and strive to follow it.

Okay, you agree that you *should* witness and that you are in an ideal profession to *do* it. Otherwise, you probably would not have picked this course. But I expect that you have felt guilty for years because you rarely or never witness through your work. You probably feel an internal conflict between the church's command to "share your faith" and your medical training that said "it's unethical to impose your personal views on patients because of your powerful position." Beyond that quandary, you may feel inadequate and question: What if my patient asks me a religious question I can't answer? And perhaps worst of all, you are pressured by time constraints, wondering: How can I start that topic when I only have a few minutes with each patient?

And the bottom-line: you just don't know *how* to witness. The word "evangelism" scares you. You envision people waving Bibles and forcing tracts on strangers. You couldn't do that. It's unprofessional, and it's just not you!

But there is still that nagging problem—Jesus *COMMANDED* us to witness. So if you're like most Christian healthcare professionals, you give mental assent to the idea, but fail to carry it out. You live a double life—at times wearing your "church face" but in your practice you just put your "professional face" on. Your fractured life causes tension and mental conflict, but you have suppressed it. You're just focused on getting through the day.

I admit that I'm twisting the knife by now. That's because I am speaking to myself. I have been that multiple personality Christian healthcare professional who desperately needed to be shaken out of my complacent routine. I have been the doctor who failed to find fulfillment in practice and had the nagging knowledge of an important missing element. I claimed that I wanted to be like the Great Physician, but deep inside I knew I was not. How could I be like Christ if I failed to address the spiritual needs of my patients?

I'm so glad I am no longer that kind of healthcare professional and you don't have to be either. The training you will receive in *Grace Prescriptions* builds on the strong foundation of CMDA's acclaimed

If the average healthcare professional sees one hundred patients a week, that translates into two hundred million opportunities to share the love of Christ every year.

Saline Solution curriculum used to train almost twenty thousand healthcare professionals around the world. Maybe you are coming to this for a refresher after attending *Saline Solution* or you may have never been exposed to a course that integrates addressing spiritual issues in a healthcare setting. Watch out. What you are about to experience will transform your life and practice. You will go to work with a whole new sense of purpose and God's presence.

You will learn that witnessing is not a formula or a tract; it is simply telling people what God is doing in your life. You will find that witnessing is not time-consuming. It is as easy as having a cup of coffee, and you can do it with each patient. Not only is it ethical, it is probably unethical not to provide for your patients' spiritual health as you care for their physical health. You will even discover that a relationship with God can have a positive impact on your patients' health. And you will learn much more, until sharing the love of Christ becomes a natural and fulfilling part of your daily life whether you are in the OR, ER, hospital, exam room, lab, or doctors' lounge.

As a bonus, your calling to medicine will be refreshed and you will find new purpose and fulfillment in practice. You will conform your routine day to the pattern of the Great Physician's, who not only healed but also dealt with the deepest longings of each individual He encountered.

The Christian Medical & Dental Associations' (CMDA) number one priority is training healthcare professionals like you to integrate their faith into their practice of healthcare. We know that outreach is God's top priority—that is why He sent His Son—so it must be ours as well. Our goal is to revitalize the twenty thousand medical and dental professionals we have trained and to educate that many more who have no spiritual ministry training to be salt in the healthcare world. If the average healthcare professional sees one hundred patients a week, that will translate into almost two hundred million opportunities to share the love of Christ every year.

After you complete the course, train others in your practice or community using the small group video series materials. We want every Christian nurse, physician, physician assistant, nurse practitioner, dentist and other healthcare practitioners to integrate their faith and have an effective ministry in their practices.

Therefore go and make disciples of all nations, baptizing them in the name of the Father and of the Son and of the Holy Spirit, and teaching them to obey everything I have commanded you. And surely I am with you always, to the very end of the age.

—Matthew 28:19-20

Though it is our priority, training healthcare professionals to witness is not all we do. CMDA has more than forty ministries "to transform healthcare professionals to transform the world." If you are not a CMDA member, I invite you to visit *www.cmda.org* and join this movement of Christian healthcare professionals determined to change the world. If you join, we will not only change the world, through CMDA, God will change *you*.

ABOUT THE AUTHORS

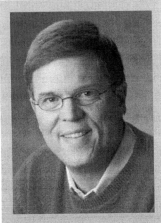

Walt Larimore, MD

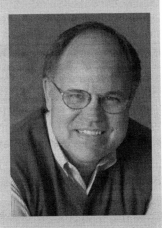

William C. Peel, ThM

Walt Larimore, MD, award-winning family physician, bestselling author and educator, has been called "one of America's best-known family physicians." He serves on the adjunct family medicine faculty of the In His Image Family Medicine Residency in Tulsa, Oklahoma, and the University of Colorado Health Sciences Center in Denver, Colorado. Dr. Larimore is a prolific author, having published 30 books, 30 medical textbook chapters and nearly 700 articles in a variety of medical journals and lay magazines. His books have garnered a number of national awards, including a Book of the Year Award from ECPA. Dr. Larimore and Barb, his sweetheart from childhood, have been married 40 years. They have two adult children, two grandchildren and a cat named Jack. Visit his website at *www.DrWalt.com*. His new daily Bible devotional, *Morning Glory, Evening Grace,* is available at *www.Devotional.DrWalt.com*.

William C. Peel, ThM, is the former director of CMDA's Paul Tournier Institute. For more than 25 years, he has helped people identify their calling and close the gap between Sunday faith and Monday work. Bill serves as founding Executive Director of the Center for Faith & Work at LeTourneau University and is an award-winning author of seven books including *Workplace Grace* and *What God Does When Men Pray*. He holds a master's degree from Dallas Theological Seminary and is a doctoral candidate at Gordon-Conwell Seminary. Bill and his wife Kathy have been married for 41 years and live in Dallas. They have three grown sons, two daughters-in-law, one granddaughter and a Border collie named Hank. For more information about Bill and the Center for Faith & Work, visit *www.centerforfaithandwork.com*.

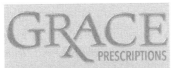

Course Objectives

At the end of this course, the health professional should:

1. Understand the relationship between spiritual health and physical / emotional / relational health.
2. Understand and ethically be able to incorporate a number of spiritual interventions into day-to-day patient care.
3. Be able to utilize a spiritual assessment, when indicated.
4. Be able to utilize faith flags, faith stories, and faith prescriptions, when indicated.
5. Understand how to utilize spiritual consults or referrals, when indicated.
6. Be able to share their personal faith story (testimony).
7. Be able to briefly share the gospel, when indicated.
8. Understand how to appropriately pray with and for patients, when indicated.
9. Be able to teach these principles to other health professionals within their influence.
10. Understand why spiritual interventions, when indicated, are appropriate and ethical in healthcare.
11. Discuss faith and apply spiritual interventions when appropriate.

Key Questions

1. Why should we, as Christian health professionals, consider incorporating our spiritual faith into our day-to-day work?
2. In other words, should we bring our spiritual profession into our vocational profession?

MODULE 1
Introduction

As a Christian in healthcare, you have an unparalleled privilege of impacting the lives of patients. You apply potent healing skills to bear on their most pressing physical, emotional, and relational needs. And as a follower of Christ, you bring an added spiritual dimension to your work that enables you to minister to the whole person. In this course, you will learn why spiritual interventions are appropriate and also develop skills to diagnose and effectively address your patients' spiritual needs.

Meet Your Colleagues

Please introduce yourself to the people in your group or at your table. Include your name, your vocation, and where you live. In one breath, tell why you entered healthcare.

NAME	VOCATION	LOCATION

Case Study

A health professional has terminal cancer and, for the first time, is facing the reality of impending death. Early in their career, the professional made an error that resulted in a patient's untimely death. Ever since then, the professional has been wracked with guilt and is now wondering how a loving God could ever offer forgiveness for such a terrible outcome. The professional is terrified of dying and desperately wants to be forgiven. If you were caring for this person, what would you do? What would you say? How would you respond?

What Do You Think?

After viewing the video, discuss the following questions:

► What did this patient want? What did he need?

► What could you have done in this situation?

11

Why We're Here

A Tremendous _____

"Therefore, if anyone is in Christ, he is a new creation; the old has gone, the new has come! All this is from God, who reconciled us to himself through Christ and gave us the ministry of reconciliation: that God was reconciling the world to himself in Christ, not counting men's sins against them. And he has committed to us the message of reconciliation. We are therefore Christ's ambassadors, as though God were making his appeal through us…"

—2 Corinthians 5:17-20

A Remarkable _____

"'Everyone who calls on the name of the Lord will be saved.' How, then, can they call on the one they have not believed in? And how can they believe in the one of whom they have not heard? And how can they hear without someone preaching to them? And how can they preach unless they are sent? As it is written, 'How beautiful are the feet of those who bring good news!'"

—Romans 10:13-15

"But in your hearts set apart Christ as Lord. Always be prepared to give an answer to everyone who asks you to give the reason for the hope that you have. But do this with gentleness and respect."

—1 Peter 3:15

A Critical _____

"I pray that you may be active in sharing your faith, so that you will have a full understanding of every good thing we have in Christ."

—Philemon 1:6

What's Ahead

Modules 2-5: We will review the latest research on the appropriateness of spiritual interventions in a clinical setting.

Module 6-8: We will investigate the basic principles involved in introducing spiritual interventions in a clinical setting.

Modules 9-12: We will familiarize you with a number of practical tools you can use to appropriately invite your patients to take a step closer to God.

Modules 13-14: We will teach you how to use the most powerful tool in your spiritual armamentarium and bring this course to a conclusion.

> In the medical profession, we do have a matchless, wonderful opportunity to meet people at times of their real need when they are ready to open up their hearts and expose their fears and worries and concerns. They will talk about their families and about eternity and the other things that are bottled up inside them. They are broken and afraid when they face a medical situation. They often are very willing to express these things, and this gives us the opportunity to present the grace of our Lord Jesus Christ.[1]
>
> —Paul Brand, MD

> No physician, sleepless and worried about a patient, can return to the hospital in the midnight hours without feeling the importance of his faith. The dim corridor is silent; the doors are closed. At the end of the corridor in the glow of the desk lamp, the nurse watches over those who sleep or lie lonely and wait. No physician entering the hospital in these quiet hours can help feeling that the medical institution of which he is part is in essence religious, that it is built on trust.
>
> No physician can fail to be proud that he is part of his patient's faith.[2]
>
> —George Crile, Jr., MD

Citations

1.   Brand, P. *Evangelism for the Medical & Dental Professions*. CMDS, ca. 1990. p.19.
2.   Crile, G. *Cancer and common sense*. Viking Press, 1955.

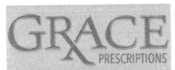

Module 2
Are Spiritual Interventions Appropriate in Clinical Care?

Key Questions
1. What spiritual interventions could a health professional consider?
2. What principles should always be applied to spiritual interventions?

It was he who gave some to be apostles, some to be prophets, some to be evangelists, and some to be pastors and teachers, to prepare God's people for works of service, so that the body of Christ may be built up.
—Ephesians 4:11-12

I pray that you may be active in sharing your faith, so that you will have a full understanding of every good thing we have in Christ.
—Philemon 1:6

"Interested clinicians and systems should learn to assess their patients' spiritual health and to provide indicated and desired spiritual intervention.

"Clinicians and health care systems should not, without compelling data to the contrary, deprive their patients of the spiritual support and comfort on which their hope, health, and well-being may hinge."[1]
—Walt Larimore, MD, et al.

Until modern times, spirituality and healthcare were inseparably linked. Only in recent times and in developed countries have these systems of healing been separated. However, current research, patient openness, and biblical precedent all suggest the importance and appropriateness of a holistic approach to quality patient care, which includes spiritual as well as medical components.

Case Study

You overhear one of your supervisors or colleagues, who is older and much more experienced, having a discussion with an elderly patient.

"Everything seems to be in good shape. We've already talked about exercise and diet, which are important in reducing health risks.

"There's also another factor research shows is highly significant and which you may want to consider. People who deepen their spiritual health may improve their ability to recover from or cope with disease. You may want to consider this as you decide how to improve your health. And, if you're interested, I can tell you about a number of spiritual treatments we could consider."

Would you have been surprised to hear something like this coming from a supervisor or colleague? Would you have thought it appropriate? Why or why not?

Read Ephesians 4:11 and Philemon 1:6. Whose responsibility is ministry according to Paul?

What are the most compelling personal reasons you see for you to be involved in caring for your patients spiritually?

How have you seen God at work in the patients with which you are interacting?

What does God seem to be up to from your perspective?

What Do We Mean by Spiritual Interventions?

There is a spectrum of "spiritual interventions" or "spiritual care" each Christian health professional can consider.

1. Ignore the connection between spirituality/religiousness and physical/emotional health.

2. Ignore your patient's religion/spirituality or lack thereof.

3. Recognize the connection between spirituality/religiousness and physical/emotional health.

---

4. Assess your patient's spirituality/religiousness.

5. Provide spiritual/religious consult/referral.

6. Provide faith flags, faith stories, and/or faith prescriptions with a patient when appropriate.

7. Pray with or for a patient.

8. Provide spiritual counseling with your patient.

Vital Protocol: When is it appropriate?

Spiritual interventions 4-8 must follow these principles:[2]

▶ _____ for the patient

▶ _____ to the patient

▶ _____ of the patient

What Is Appropriate? (for group discussion)

NOTE: A far more detailed PowerPoint presentation of this topic is available from CMDA for use in self-study or for teaching:

- Are Spiritual Interventions Appropriate in Clinical Care? What Does the Research Say?

Citations

1. Larimore, WL, Parker, M, Crowther, M. Should clinicians incorporate positive spirituality into their practices? What does the evidence say? (Review). *Annals of Behavioral Medicine* 2002;24(1):69-73.
2. Gostin, LO. Informed Consent, Cultural Sensitivity, and Respect for Persons. *JAMA* 1995;274(10):844-845.

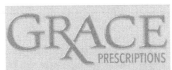

The Case for Spiritual Interventions

While spiritual interventions in clinical care have come under fire from certain circles in the academic world, the research findings, patient desire, and common sense all argue for the inclusion of an appropriate spiritual component. Not only is there no evidence that such therapy is harmful, but the research clearly supports the association of positive spirituality to physical, emotional, and spiritual health.

Case Study

Jane is a patient you are seeing for the first time. As you are taking her history, she tells you she is transferring from the care of another health professional.

She says, "I was very offended by the man. First of all, he had all this freaky religious art and Scripture verses all over the place. Then, when we began to talk, he asked me if I had ever attended religious services. I told him, in no uncertain terms, that it was none of his business. I think this shocked him. But then he had the gall to ask me if I knew where I would spend eternity if I were to die that night. I blew up, and I told him where I thought he could go before I stormed out of the office." Then Jane is quiet for a moment before saying, "He really scared me. I'll never go to a religious provider again. Everyone knows that you don't talk about politics or religion—particularly in healthcare!"

The Case against Spiritual Interventions

Academic Voices in Opposition

▶ Sloan, RP, et al. Religion, spirituality, and medicine. *Lancet* 1999;353:664-667.[8]

▶ Sloan, RP, et al. Should physicians prescribe religious activities? *New England Journal of Medicine* 2000;342:1913-1916.[9]

▶ Sloan, RP, Bagiella, E. Data without a prayer. *Archives of Internal Medicine* 2000;160:1870.[10]

▶ Sloan, RP, Bagiella, E. Spirituality and Medical Practice: A Look at the Evidence. *American Family Physician* 2001;63:33-35.[11]

▶ Sloan, RP, Bagiella, E. Claims about religious involvement and health outcomes. *Annals of Behavioral Medicine* 2002(Winter);24(1):14-21.[1]

Sloan's Conclusion

Because of weak data support and the potential danger involved, health professionals should not practice spiritual interventions.

The Case for Spiritual Intervention

1. Is the data weak?

In addressing this criticism, even in 2001, the authors of the *Oxford University Handbook of Religion and Health* concluded, "We simply disagree."[2]

The quantity of data is _____.

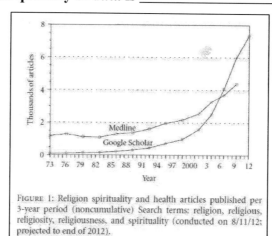

FIGURE 1: Religion spirituality and health articles published per 3-year period (noncumulative) Search terms: religion, religious, religiosity, religiousness, and spirituality (conducted on 8/11/12; projected to end of 2012).

Koenig, HG. Review Article: Religion, Spirituality, and Health: The Research and Clinical Implications. *ISRN Psychiatry*. Dec 16, 2012:278730.

As seen in the graph above, the volume of research on religion/spirituality R/S and health has dramatically increased since the mid-1990s. About 50% of these articles are original research (with quantitative data), while the other 50% are qualitative reports, opinion pieces, reviews, or commentaries.

In 2002, Walt Larimore, MD, and his colleagues listed nearly forty major systematic reviews that examined the R/S-health connection and reported a positive risk-benefit ratio.[4] They found that:

▶ The _____ outweigh the risks.

"Dozens of systematic reviews have all concluded that in the vast majority of patients the apparent benefits of intrinsic religious belief and practice outweigh the risks."[4]

▶ The evidence against spiritual intervention is not _____.

"Most of the rhetoric decrying the incorporation of basic and positive spiritual care into clinical practice is not based on reliable evidence. There is most frequently a positive association between positive spirituality and (1) mental health, (2) physical health, and (3) wellbeing."[4]

▶ Evidence _____ basic spiritual interventions.

"The evidence to date demonstrates trained or experienced clinicians should encourage positive spirituality with their patients and that there is no evidence that such therapy is, in general, harmful."[4]

There are, in fact, thousands of quantitative original data-based research reports examining relationships between R/S (religion/spirituality) and health ... that have been published in peer-reviewed journals in medicine, nursing, social work, rehabilitation, social sciences, counseling, psychology, psychiatry, public health, demography, economics, law, and religion.[3]

—Oxford Handbook of Religion and Health

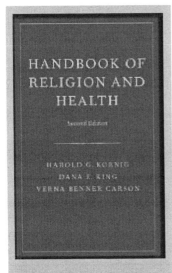

The data is of _____ quality.

In a 2012 systematic review that summarized the massive *Oxford University Handbook of Religion and Health*,[3] Harold Koenig, MD, a psychiatrist at Duke University, reported that a large majority of the 3,300 studies he reviewed were rated "higher quality" (Cooper scores 7-10 out of 10).[5]

> "Despite the negative views and opinions held by many mental health professionals, research examining religion, spirituality, and health has been rapidly expanding—and most of it is occurring outside the field of psychiatry."[5]

> "These reports have been published in peer-reviewed journals in medicine, nursing, social work, rehabilitation, social sciences, counseling, psychology, psychiatry, public health, demography, economics, and religion. The majority of studies report significant relationships between R/S and better health."[5]

2. Do we need to wait for randomized clinical trials?

▶ We _____ wait for randomized clinical trials to practice healthcare. This argument, if applied to healthcare uniformly, would bring healthcare to a halt.[4]

> "Therapies that are inexpensive, easy to apply, desired by the patient, that have minimal risk of harm, and appear to be helpful (even based upon uncontrolled or anecdotal data), are considered reasonable to most clinicians.

> "However, it would be unwise to utilize any therapy, without controlled data, that has a high probability of being harmful."[4]
>
> —Walt Larimore, MD, et al.

3. Are spiritual interventions beyond the domain of practice?

▶ All factors that influence health can and, when appropriate, *should be* addressed in providing evidence-based, high-quality healthcare.

▶ Health professionals often offer "non-medical" advice.[4]

> "Many healthcare professionals ... when asked about marriage versus cohabitation, for example, would be very comfortable recommending the former. ... when asked about marital versus non-marital sex by a teen, most would be very comfortable recommending the former ... based upon the data."[4]
>
> —Walt Larimore, MD, et al

4. Is spiritual intervention coercive?

► Spiritual care or interventions _____
coercive, especially if not data-driven and not administered with
patient permission ... However, data-based recommendations on
other social issues are not viewed as coercive. Many are now
considered quality healthcare.[4]

"Healthcare professionals, familiar with the social science healthcare data,
often make specific recommendations about a number of social health issues,
including, but not limited to, number of sexual partners, alcohol/tobacco/drug
use, firearms in the home, seat belt use, etc."[4]

—Walt Larimore, MD, et al.

5. Does spiritual intervention cause harm?

► Any intervention could _____
cause harm. However, to date, there is no evidence to support this
concern for spiritual care. Furthermore, patients with negative
spiritual beliefs that are not addressed may have a significantly
increased morbidity and mortality.[4]

For example, in one longitudinal cohort study of hospitalized
patients, those who: (1) wondered whether God had abandoned
them, (2) questioned God's love for them, (3) decided the devil
made this happen, OR (4) felt punished by God for their lack of
devotion ... experienced 16% to 28% higher mortality during a
two-year period following hospital discharge.[6]

6. Does spiritual intervention risk dualism toward patients?

► Classes of patients are a _____.
Patients make the decisions, not health professionals.[4]

"Classes of patients, like smokers and non-smokers, are created by the patient
and not by us. Our job is to use our patient's history to recognize the
differences, assess the risks, and make data-based recommendations."[4]

—Walt Larimore, MD, et al.

► By respectfully _____
spiritual topics with patients who are open, we are much more
likely to help than harm.[4]

"Professional problems can occur when well-meaning physicians 'faith-push' a
patient opposed to discussing religion ... However, rather than ignoring faith
completely with all patients, most of whom want to discuss it, physicians
might ask a question to discern who would like to pursue it and who would
rather not."[12]

—Stephen G. Post, PhD

We believe that there are sufficient, research-based reasons for clinicians to provide basic spiritual interventions.[4]
—Walt Larimore, MD, et al.

7. Is spiritual intervention premature?

► Larimore, et al., wrote, "Most of the rhetoric decrying the incorporation of basic and positive spiritual care into clinical practice is _____ based on reliable evidence."[4]

► In his systematic review, Koenig wrote, "There are many practical reasons why addressing spiritual issues in clinical practice is important."[5]

► Larimore, et al., cite six evidence-based reasons why spiritual interventions in clinical care are not premature:[4]

1. A Positive _____

   "There is frequently a positive association between positive spirituality and (1) mental health, (2) physical health, and (3) wellbeing."[4]

2. Patient _____

   "Most patients desire to be offered basic spiritual care by their clinicians."[4]

3. Patient _____

   "Most patients censure our professions for ignoring their spiritual needs."[4]

4. Clinicians _____

   "Most clinicians believe that spiritual interventions would help their patients but have little training in providing basic spiritual assessment or care."[4]

5. Professional _____

   "Professional associations and educational institutions are beginning to provide learners and clinicians information on how to incorporate spirituality and practice."[4]

6. Anecdotal _____

   "Anecdotal evidence indicates that clinicians having received such training find it immediately helpful and do apply it to their practice."[4]

Conclusion

"The evidence to date demonstrates clinicians should encourage positive spirituality with their patients and that there is no evidence that such therapy is, in general, harmful."[4]

—Walt Larimore, MD, et al.

What is positive spirituality?
Positive spirituality involves a growing, internalized personal relationship with the sacred or transcendent that is:
1. not bound by race, ethnicity, economics, or class;
2. promotes the wellness and welfare of self and others; and
3. results in the "fruit" of love, joy, peace, patience, kindness, goodness, faithfulness, gentleness, and self-control.[4]
—Walt Larimore, MD, et al.

19

The research findings, a desire to provide high-quality care, and simply common sense, all underscore the need to integrate spirituality into patient care.[5]
—Harold Koenig, MD

"Nothing in life is more wonderful than faith ... the one great moving force which we can neither weigh in the balance nor test in the crucible ... mysterious, indefinable, known only by its effects, faith pours out an unfailing stream of energy while abating neither jot nor tittle of its potence."[7]
—Sir William Osler, MD

NOTE: Two far more detailed PowerPoint presentations are available from CMDA for use in self-study or teaching:
- What is the Connection between Spirituality / Religiousness and Physical / Emotional Health? What Does the Research Say?
- Are Spiritual Interventions Appropriate in Clinical Care? What Does the Research Say?

Summary

"Until there is evidence of harm from a clinician's provision of either basic spiritual care or a spiritually sensitive practice, interested clinicians and systems should learn to assess their patients' spiritual health and to provide indicated and desired spiritual intervention.[4]

"It is highly ethical for healthcare professionals (and even healthcare systems) to assess their patients' spiritual health and needs, and to provide indicated and desired spiritual interventions.[4]

"Clinicians and healthcare systems should not, without compelling data to the contrary, deprive their patients of the spiritual support and comfort on which their hope, health, and wellbeing may hinge."[4]

—Walt Larimore, MD, et al.

"At stake is the health and wellbeing of our patients and satisfaction that we as healthcare providers experience in delivering care that addresses the whole person—body, mind, and spirit."[5]

—Harold Koenig, MD

Group Discussion

Discuss the following questions in your group:

▸ Have you personally encountered resistance to including spiritual care in a clinical setting?

▸ In your opinion, what is the strongest argument against spiritual care?

▸ In your opinion, what is the strongest argument for spiritual care?

Citations

1. Sloan, RP, Bagiella, E. Claims about religious involvement and health outcomes. *Annals of Behavioral Medicine* 2002(Winter);24(1):14-21.
2. Koenig, HG, McCullogh, ME, Larson, DB. *Handbook of Religion and Health.* Oxford University Press, 2001.
3. Koenig, H, King, D, Carson, VB. *Handbook of Religion and Health – Second Edition.* Oxford University Press, 2012.
4. Larimore, WL, Parker, M, Crowther, M. Should clinicians incorporate positive spirituality into their practices? What does the evidence say? (Review) *Annals of Behavioral Medicine* 2002;24(1):69-73.
5. Koenig, HG. Review Article: Religion, Spirituality, and Health: The Research and Clinical Implications. *ISRN Psychiatry*. Dec 16, 2012:278730.
6. Pargament, K, et al. Religious struggle as a predictor of mortality among medically ill elderly patients: a two-year longitudinal study. *Archives of Internal Medicine*. 2001;161:1881-1885.
7. Osler, W. *The Faith That Heals*. Br Med J 1910(Jun 18);1(2581):1470-1472.
8. Sloan, RP, et al. Religion, spirituality, and medicine. *Lancet* 1999;353:664-667.
9. Sloan, RP, et al. Should physicians prescribe religious activities? *New England Journal of Medicine* 2000;342:1913-1916.
10. Sloan, RP, Bagiella E. Data without a prayer. *Archives of Internal Medicine* 2000;160(12):1870-1871.
11. Sloan, RP, Bagiella E. Spirituality and Medical Practice: A Look at the Evidence. *American Family Physician* 2001;63:33-5
12. Post, SG. Ethical Aspects of Religion in Healthcare. *Mind/Body Medicine: A Journal of Clinical Behavioral Medicine*. 1996;2(1):44-48.

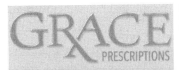

Module 4
The Biblical and Ethical Case for Spiritual Care

Key Questions
1. What is the relationship of physical and spiritual health from a biblical perspective?
2. What is the rebuttal to common ethical arguments made against providing spiritual care?

News about him spread all over Syria, and people brought to him all who were ill with various diseases, those suffering severe pain, the demon-possessed, those having seizures, and the paralyzed, and he healed them.
—Matthew 4:24

Jesus loves this man so much, He gives him, first, not what he came for, but what he longed for—that which would truly satisfy: spiritual wholeness through a relationship with God.

The Bible refuses to reduce human sickness, disease, and suffering to a simplistic cause. It sees human misery as complex, multidimensional, interrelated—and refuses to separate physical suffering and spiritual need. If this perspective is accurate, then it presents a significant ethical dilemma to health professionals, particularly Christians, who are reluctant to provide spiritual care for their patients.

Case Study: Jesus Heals a Paralyzed Man

Read Mark 2:1-12 in your group.

Mark 2:1-12

A few days later, when Jesus again entered Capernaum, the people heard that he had come home. So many gathered that there was no room left, not even outside the door, and he preached the word to them.

Some men came, bringing to him a paralytic, carried by four of them. Since they could not get him to Jesus because of the crowd, they made an opening in the roof above Jesus and, after digging through it, lowered the mat the paralyzed man was lying on. When Jesus saw their faith, he said to the paralytic, "Son, your sins are forgiven."

Now some teachers of the law were sitting there, thinking to themselves, "Why does this fellow talk like that? He's blaspheming! Who can forgive sins but God alone?"

Immediately Jesus knew in his spirit that this was what they were thinking in their hearts, and he said to them, "Why are you thinking these things? Which is easier: to say to the paralytic, 'Your sins are forgiven,' or to say, 'Get up, take your mat and walk'? But that you may know that the Son of Man has authority on earth to forgive sins...." He said to the paralytic, "I tell you, get up, take your mat and go home." He got up, took his mat and walked out in full view of them all.

This amazed everyone and they praised God, saying, "We have never seen anything like this!"

Grand Rounds with the Great Physician[1]

Jesus saw a key relationship between spiritual and physical health. In the healing of the paralyzed man in Mark 2:1-12, faith, forgiveness, and physical healing are all important parts of the work of the Great Physician. Note three things:

1. Why was this man brought to Jesus?

He had a _____ need.

He also had an _____ need.

2. What did he need most from Jesus?

Jesus looks right past the reason he came to his real need and says, "Son, your sins are forgiven." If one doesn't see the relationship between physical, emotional, and spiritual heath, Jesus' response borders on being a cruel joke. But this was no joke to Jesus.

The main problem in a person's life is never suffering. It's _____ from God.

Jesus loves this man too much to give him what he came for without giving him what he _____ for.

Delivering physical healing without spiritual healing _____ gets to the root of the problem.

The _____ we long for can't be obtained through procedures, drugs, or therapies.

3. What can we learn from the Great Physician's example?

It is obvious from Jesus' ministry that He saw a key relationship between spiritual and physical health. We see three important lessons to learn from Jesus' example.

1. Your patients' _____ need is spiritual, not physical, healing.

2. Physical, spiritual, and emotional needs can be appropriately treated _____ when the opportunity arises.

3. Health professionals should be just as _____ to patients' spiritual needs as they are of their physical needs and ready and willing to treat the whole person.

Men and women remain broken and unsatisfied because the roots of discontent of the human heart go far deeper than physical healing can touch. The wholeness we long for can't be obtained through procedures, drugs, or therapies alone.

Ultimately we treat patients' spiritual needs not because it may enhance their physical health but because we love them in Jesus' name and care about them as Jesus does.

Ethical Considerations

Health professionals must always respect the patient's rights to:
- Autonomy in beliefs and practices
- Confidentiality
- Privacy

1. **Patients come for medical, not _____, help, BUT ...**

   ▶ The cause of their physical problems may have spiritual or emotional roots.

   ▶ God may have directed them to you for spiritual reasons.

   ▶ Jesus combined the physical and spiritual even when people came to Him for only physical healing.

2. **It is taking advantage of a patient's _____, BUT ...**

   ▶ None of us would have come to Christ without a sense of vulnerability.

   ▶ Everyone is vulnerable 24 hours a day.

   ▶ A full dose of Jesus Christ is the only cure for the ultimate vulnerability of every sinful person.

3. **If you're trying to use a _____, you can't focus on good healthcare, BUT ...**

   ▶ This dichotomous view brings only a portion of who you are to only a portion of your patient's needs.

   ▶ Jesus provides an example of a more holistic view of treating disease.

   ▶ Consider the ethical problem of withholding information of benefit to your patient.

   ▶ Can you provide quality care and never address the spiritual?

Take an Eternal Perspective

This is a divine _____.

I need to ask, _____?

25

> Therefore, as God's chosen people, holy and dearly loved, clothe yourselves with compassion, kindness, humility, gentleness and patience. Bear with each other and forgive whatever grievances you may have against one another. Forgive as the Lord forgave you. And over all these virtues put on love, which binds them all together in perfect unity.
> —Colossians 3:12-14

Assess Your _____.

- ▶ Your overriding goal should be: How can I express the <u>love</u> of Christ to this patient?

- ▶ Approaching patients with an agenda other than to love and serve them in Jesus' name violates ethical and biblical standards.

Think _____.

- ▶ It would be unethical not to offer healthcare treatment which is indicated and which you are capable of giving.

- ▶ How much more unethical to withhold the cure for the sickness of the soul!

Discuss the following question in your group:

What is the strongest argument for including spiritual care in your practice?

What is the strongest argument for excluding spiritual care in your practice?

Citations

1. Keller, TJ. "The Healing of Forgiveness." From the series: *King's Cross: The Gospel of Mark, Part 1: The Coming of the King.* February 12, 2006. Available at http://sermons.redeemer.com/store/

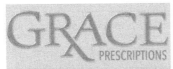

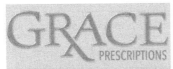

Module 5
The Importance of a Spiritual History to Quality Patient Care

Key Questions
1. Why is a spiritual history in the clinical practice of healthcare appropriate?
2. What are the benefits of a spiritual history for the patient and the health professional in clinical practice?
3. What spiritual history questions would be appropriate for me to use with my patients?

Current research, patient openness, evidence-based clinical guidelines, and biblical precedent all suggest the importance and appropriateness of a holistic approach to quality patient care—which includes a spiritual assessment for many, if not most, patients.

Case Study

Mrs. Jones, a 25-year-old woman, was brought to the ER of your hospital by ambulance with extremely heavy vaginal bleeding one week after giving birth to her first child. You are unable to stop the bleeding with medications. The patient has lost an estimated two-thirds of her blood supply; so you decide to place a central line, give her IV fluids, and order blood for an immediate transfusion.

The blood is ordered, but takes longer than usual to arrive. The patient becomes even more hypotensive, weak, and tachycardic. In addition, she becomes confused. The blood finally arrives, but you decide that the patient is not competent to sign the consent. You ask the nurse to have any family in the waiting room sign the consent.

The nurse returns to tell you that there is no family. You look on the chart for a spiritual history, but find it was not filled out, even though it is both yours and the hospital's policy to obtain one on every admission.

You order the transfusion given. When the patient's sister, her only living adult relative, arrives, you meet her and explain the situation.

The sister pales as she tells you her sister and the entire family are Jehovah's Witnesses, and they will sue you, the hospital, and "everyone in sight" for giving her blood.

If the patient's spiritual history had been complete, how might that have changed this case?

The Purpose of Spiritual History

According to Koenig,[1] the purpose of a spiritual history is to learn:

1. The patient's religious background,

2. The role that religious or spiritual beliefs or practices play in coping with illness (or causing distress),

3. Beliefs that may influence or conflict with decisions about medical care,

4. The patient's level of participation in a spiritual community and whether the community is supportive, and

5. Any spiritual needs that might be present.

Five Evidence-Based Reasons to Take a Spiritual History

1. Patient _____

"With 70% of the population viewing religious commitment as a central life factor …

- ▶ Treatment approaches devoid of spiritual sensitivity may provide an alien values framework.

- ▶ A majority of the population probably prefers an orientation … that is sympathetic, or at least sensitive, to a spiritual perspective."[4]

"In general, the public appears to view and value spirituality …

- ▶ as a central factor of life when facing illness

- ▶ and desires healthcare professionals to inquire about beliefs that are important to them."[6]

2. Patient _____

Of studies reporting relationships between R/S (religion/spirituality) and mental or physical health:

- ▶ ~1,600 (~70%) of the studies reported positive relationships,

- ▶ ~500 (~22%) of the studies reported no or mixed relationships, and

- ▶ ~200 (~9%) of the studies reported negative relationships (4% of mental health studies; 8.5% of physical health studies).

- ▶ ~1,400 (~61%) of these studies were rated high or higher quality studies (greater than 7/10 on the Cooper Rating Scale).[8]

28

3. Identification of _____

There is an inverse association between faith and morbidity and mortality of various types.[1,8,9] Religious struggles can predict mortality.

> Men and women who experience a religious struggle with their illness appear to be at increased risk of death, even after controlling for baseline health, mental health status, and demographic factors.[7]
> —Ken Pargament, PhD, et al.

► Higher religious struggle scores are predictive of 6% greater risk of mortality (P = 0.02).

► Patients who felt alienated from or unloved by God or attributed their illnesses to the devil were associated with a 16% to 28% increase in risk of dying during the two-year follow-up period.[7]

"Such patients may, without their doctor's encouragement, refuse to speak with clergy because they are angry with God and have cut themselves off from this source of support."[10]

4. May _____ Healthcare

In a large systematic review of the literature examining the association of religious commitment and health status, the authors conclude:

> The available data suggest that practitioners who make several small changes in how patients' religious commitments are broached in clinical practice may enhance healthcare outcomes.[9]
> —Dale Matthews, MD

"The empirical literature from epidemiological and clinical studies regarding the relationship between religious factors and physical and mental health status in the areas of prevention, coping, and recovery was reviewed.

A large proportion of published empirical data suggest that religious commitment plays a beneficial role in ...

► preventing mental/physical illness

► improving how people cope with mental and physical illness

► facilitating recovery from illness."[9]

5. Considered a _____

A growing number of healthcare groups are calling for greater concern for spiritual issues in the assessment and treatment of patients.

> Today, nearly 90% of medical schools (and many nursing schools) in the U.S. include something about R/S (religion/spirituality) in their curricula and this is also true to a lesser extent in the United Kingdom and Brazil.[1]
> —Harold Koenig, MD

► Many professional organizations call for greater sensitivity and training of clinicians concerning the management of R/S issues in the assessment and treatment of patients.[15]

► A spiritual history is required by the Joint Commission for "patients cared for in hospitals or nursing homes, or by a home health agency" and "should, at a minimum, determine the patient's denomination, beliefs, and what spiritual practices are important to them."[23]

► "This information would assist in determining the impact of spirituality, if any, on the care and/or services being provided and will identify if any further assessment is needed."[23]

Which of these options seem most appropriate for your practice?

You may want to pick and choose questions from among different templates.

Either way, the best questions are the ones you'll actually begin to use in clinical practice.

Nine Published Assessment Instruments

Both religious and non-religious health professionals can ethically include a spiritual assessment in their care.

Open Invite[13]

The Open Invite is a patient-focused approach to encouraging a spiritual dialogue. It is structured to allow patients to speak further and to allow those who are not so inclined to easily opt out.

- First, it reminds health professionals that their role is to open the door to conversation and invite (never require) patients to discuss their spiritual beliefs or needs.

- Second, it suggests health professionals use a mnemonic for asking several questions to broach the topic of spirituality.

- Questions may be similar to those used in the FICA, HOPE, or GOD mnemonics, listed below, or may be customized.

Open (the door to spiritual conversation):

- May I ask your faith background?

- Do you have a spiritual or faith preference?

Invite (the patient to discuss spiritual needs using one of the mnemonics listed below or one or more of these questions):

- Do you feel that your spiritual health is affecting your physical health?

- Does your spirituality impact the health decisions you make?

- Is there a way in which you would like for me to account for your spirituality in your care?

- Is there a way we can provide spiritual support?

- Are there resources in your faith community that you would like for me to help mobilize?

FICA

The FICA Spiritual History Tool uses an acronym to guide health professionals through a series of questions designed to elicit patient spirituality and its potential effect on healthcare.

Starting with queries about faith and belief, it proceeds to ask about their importance to the patient, the patient's community of faith, and how the patient wishes the professional to address spirituality in his or her care.[14,15]

HOPE

These questions lead the health professional from general concepts to specific applications by asking about patients' sources of hope and meaning, whether they belong to an organized religion, their personal spirituality and practices, and what effect their spirituality may have on medical care and end-of-life decisions.[16]

FICA Spiritual History[14,15]

F = Faith. Do you have spiritual beliefs that help you cope? If the patient responds "no," consider asking: What gives your life meaning or hope?

I = Importance. Have your beliefs influenced how you take care of yourself in this illness?

C = Community. Are you part of a spiritual community? Is this of support to you? If so, how?

A = Address. How would you like me to address these issues in your healthcare? Are there any spiritual resources you might need?

HOPE Spiritual History[16]

H = Hope. What sources of hope, strength, comfort, meaning, peace, love, and connection do you have? What do you hold on to during difficult times?

O = Organized religion. Are you part of a religious or spiritual community? Does it help you? If so, how?

P = Personal spirituality or practices. Do you have personal religious or spiritual beliefs? What aspects of your spirituality or spiritual practices do you find most helpful?

E = Effects on care. Is there anything I can do to help you access the spiritual resources that usually help you? Are there any specific practices or restrictions I should know about in providing your medical care?

SPIRITual History[17]

S = Spiritual belief system. Do you have a formal religious affiliation? Do you have a spiritual life that is important to you?

P = Personal spirituality. In what ways is your religion or spirituality meaningful to you?

I = Integration with faith community. Do you participate in a faith community? What support does this group give you?

R = Ritualized practices and restrictions. What specific lifestyle activities or practices does your religion/spirituality encourage?

I = Implications for medical practice. What aspects of your R/S would you like me to keep in mind as I care for you?

T = Terminal events planning. Will your R/S influence your end-of-life decisions?

FAITH Spiritual History[18]

F = Faith. Do you have a spiritual faith or religion that is important to you?

A = Apply. How do your beliefs apply to your health?

I = Involved. Are you involved in a faith community?

T = Treatment. How do your spiritual views affect your views about treatment?

H = Help. How can I help you with any spiritual concerns?

CSI-MEMO Spiritual History[19]

CS = Comfort/Stress. Do your R/S beliefs provide comfort or are they a source of stress?

I = Influence. Do you have R/S beliefs that might influence your medical decisions?

MEM = Member. Are you a member of an R/S community and is it supportive to you?

O = Other. Do you have other spiritual needs you'd like someone to address?

ACP/ASIM Spiritual History[20]

1. Is faith (religion, spirituality) important to you in this illness?
2. Has faith been important to you at other times in your life?
3. Do you have someone to talk to about spiritual matters?
4. Would you like to explore religious matters with someone?

Larson Spiritual History[21]

1. Do you attend religious services? If so, how often do you generally attend?

2. Aside from attending religious services, would you say that religion is important to you?

3. Do you pray? If so, how frequently?

GOD Questions[21]

G = God. Is God, spirituality, religion, or spiritual faith important to you?

O = Others. Do you meet with others in religious or spiritual community? If so, how often? How do you integrate with your faith community?

D = Do. What can I do to assist you in incorporating your spiritual or religious faith into your medical care? Or, is there anything I can do to encourage your faith? May I pray with or for you?

While Assessing Spiritual Needs[13]

When spiritual needs have been identified …

Listen compassionately[28]

▶ Regardless of whether patients are devout in their spiritual traditions, their beliefs are important to them.

▶ By listening, even for just a few seconds, the health professional signals his or her care for their patients and recognition of this dimension of their lives.

Respect and Clarify[1]

▶ The religious or spiritual beliefs of patients uncovered during the spiritual history should always be respected.

▶ Even if beliefs conflict with the medical treatment plan or seem bizarre or pathological, the health professional should not challenge those beliefs (at least not initially), but rather take a neutral posture and ask the patient questions to obtain a better understanding of the beliefs.

Remember to Document[1,13]

▶ Always document your spiritual assessment and your patient's openness to discussing the topic.

▶ You may find this information helpful when readdressing the subject in the future.

▶ This documentation also helps meet any regulatory requirements for conducting a spiritual assessment.

Learn how different traditions and practices may affect standard medical practice.[1,13]

Empathetic listening may be all the support a patient requires.[13]
—Aaron Saquil, MD, et al.

Challenging patients' religious/spiritual beliefs (at least initially) is almost always followed by resistance from the patient, or quiet noncompliance with the medical plan.[1]
—Harold Koenig, MD

Resource
A brief description of beliefs and practices for health professionals related to birth, contraception, diet, death, and organ donation is provided in Citation 23.

NOTE: Two far more detailed PowerPoint presentations are available from CMDA for use in self-study or teaching:

- What is the Connection between Spirituality / Religiousness and Physical / Emotional Health? What Does the Research Say?
- The Importance of a Spiritual History to Quality Patience Card. Evidence-Based Recommendations.

Summary

According to Saquile, et al., "Assessing and integrating patient spirituality into the healthcare encounter can build trust and rapport, broadening the physician-patient relationship and increasing its effectiveness."[13]

Most of all, the spiritual history allows us, as followers of Jesus and as Christian health professionals, to find out where our patients are in their spiritual journeys.

It allows us to see if God is already at work in their lives and join Him there in His work.

Demonstration

Take the spiritual history of an audience member.

Citations

1. Koenig, HG. Religion, Spirituality, and Health: The Research and Clinical Implications. *ISRN Psychiatry*. 2012;Article ID 278730.
2. MacLean, CD, Susi, B, Phifer, N, et al. Patient Preference for Physician Discussion and Practice of Spirituality. Results From a Multicenter Patient Survey. *Journal of General Internal Medicine*. 2003(Jan);18(1):38–43.
3. Matthews, DA. Quoted in: Sabom, M. *Light and Death*. Grand Rapids: Zondervan Publisher. 1998.
4. Bergin, AE, Jensen, JP. Religiosity of psychotherapists: A national survey. *Psychotherapy: Theory, Research, Practice, Training*. 1990;27(1):3-7.
5. Levin, JS, Vanderpool, HY. Is frequent religious attendance really conducive to better health? Toward an epidemiology of religion. *Social Science and Medicine*. 1987;24(7):589-600.
6. Hatch, RL, Burg, MA, Naberhaus, DS, et al. The Spiritual Involvement and Beliefs Scale. Development and testing of a new instrument. *Journal of Family Practice*. 1998(Jun);46(6):476-486.
7. Pargament, K, Koenig, HG, Tarakeshwar, N, et al. Religious struggle as a predictor of mortality among medically ill elderly patients: a two-year longitudinal study. *Archives of Internal Medicine*. 2001(Aug);161(15):1881-1885.
8. Koenig, HG, King, DE, Carson, VB. *Handbook of Religion and Health – Second Edition*. Oxford University Press, 2012.
9. Matthews, DA, McCullough, ME, Larson, DB, et al. Religious commitment and health status: A review of the research and implications for family medicine. *Archives of Family Medicine*. 1998(Mar);7(2):118-124.
10. Koenig, HG. An 83-Year-Old Woman With Chronic Illness and Strong Religious Beliefs. *JAMA*. 2002;288(4):487-493.
11. Sloan, RP. *Blind Faith: The Unholy Alliance of Religion and Medicine*. St. Martin's Press, 2006.
12. Larimore, WL, Parker, M, Crowther, M. Should clinicians incorporate positive spirituality into their practices? What does the evidence say? (Review) *Annals of Behavioral Medicine*. 2002(Feb);24(1):69-73.
13. Saguil, A, Phelps, K. The Spiritual Assessment. *American Family Physician*. 2012(Sep 15);86(6):546-50.
14. Borneman, T, Ferrell, B, Puchalski, CM. Evaluation of the FICA Tool for Spiritual Assessment. *Journal of Pain and Symptom Management*. 2010(Aug);40(2):163-73.
15. Puchalski, CM. Taking a Spiritual History: FICA. *Spirituality and Medicine Connection*. 1999:3:1.
16. Anandarahah, G, Hight, E. Spirituality and Medical Practice: Using the HOPE Questions as a Practical Tool for Spiritual Assessment. *American Family Physician*. 2001(Jan);63(1):81-89.
17. Maugans, TA. The SPIRITual History. *Archives of Family Medicine*. 1996(Jan);5(1):11-16.
18. King, DE. Spirituality and Medicine. In Mengal, MB, Holleman, WL, Fields, SA (eds). *Fundamentals of Clinical Practice: A Textbook on the Patient, Doctor, and Society*, (Plenum, 2002):651-659.
19. Koenig, HG. An 83-Year-Old Woman With Chronic Illness and Strong Religious Beliefs. *JAMA*. 2002;288(4):487-493.
20. Lo, B, Quill, T, Tulsky, J. Discussing palliative care with patients. ACP-ASIM End-of-Life Care Consensus Panel. American College of Physicians-American Society of Internal Medicine. *Annals of Internal Medicine* 1999(May 4);130(9):744-749.
21. Larimore, W, Peel, WC. *The Saline Solution: Sharing Christ in a Busy Practice*. Christian Medical & Dental Associations, 2000.
22. Post, SG. "Ethical Aspects of Religion in Healthcare." *Mind/Body Medicine: A Journal of Clinical Behavioral Medicine*. 1996;2(1):44-48.
23. Koenig, HG. Information on specific religions. In: *Spirituality in Patient Care. Why, How, When, and What. Second Edition*, (Templeton Press, 2007):188–227.

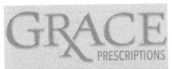

Module 6
Understanding the Barriers to Spiritual Care

Key Questions

1. How do people most frequently come to Christ?
2. What are some of the steps people take in their faith journey to trusting Christ?
3. What are some of the common barriers people face in trusting Christ?
4. What is spiritual therapy?

The health professional/patient relationship presents significant opportunities for spiritual care. However, barriers exist for both health professionals and patients. Understanding these barriers is the first step to helping patients take the next step toward a healthy relationship with God.

Case Study

People often have developed some strong visions of what it would be like to bring their faith into their work environment. After watching the video, discuss in your group:

When you think of evangelism, *what* comes to mind? Something positive or negative?

How often do faith conversations occur in your practice?

What barriers exist that make faith conversations difficult?

How Do People Come to Christ?[1]

More than 42,000 people over a 20-year period were asked the question, "What or who was responsible for your coming to Christ and your church?"

YOUR GUESS		RESEARCH
_____	Special Need	_____
_____	Walk-ins	_____
_____	Pastor	_____
_____	Church Program	_____
_____	Visitation	_____
_____	Sunday School	_____
_____	Evangelistic crusade/TV	_____
_____	Friend or relative	_____

Group Discussion

How did you come to Christ?

Why are relationships so important to spiritual influence?

According to Win and Charles Arn of Church Growth, Inc., webs of common kinship (the larger family), common friendship (friends and neighbors), and common associates (work associates and people with common interests or recreational pursuits) are still the paths most people follow in becoming Christians today.[2]

Our job is to find out what the Spirit is doing in a person's life and join Him there.

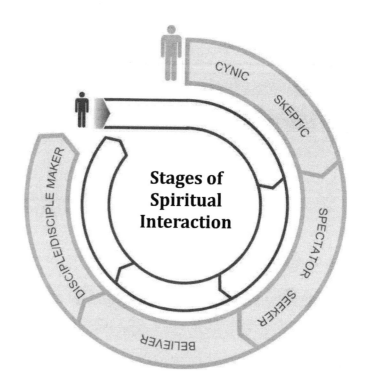

Stages of Spiritual Interaction

THE FAITH JOURNEY

When someone comes to Christ, it is never just an event. Even though we all start at different places, it is always a journey, a process. What often looks like one major choice is really the result of a multitude of small, incremental decisions as a person faces the barriers to faith.

Micro-Steps of Faith

+5 Chooses to live by faith
+4 Makes Christ-like choices
+3 Chooses to share his/her faith
+2 Joins in Christian community
+1 Assimilates God's Word

0 Trusts in Christ

-1 Turns from self-trust
-2 Sees Jesus as the answer
-3 Recognizes his/her need of Christ
-4 Considers the truth of the gospel
-5 Understands the implications of the gospel

-6 Recognizes the Bible may have answers
-7 Aware of the gospel
-8 Looks positively at the Bible

-9 Still thinks the Bible is unreliable or regressive
-10 Comes to like you even though you're a Christian
-11 Recognizes a difference in you

-12 Aware that you are a Christian
-13 Avoids the truth
-14 Hostile to the truth and Christians

DISCIPLE-MAKER	
DISCIPLE	
BELIEVER	
SEEKER	
SPECTATOR	
SKEPTIC	
CYNIC	

Then he told them many things in parables, saying: "A farmer went out to sow his seed. As he was scattering the seed, some fell along the **path**, and the **birds** came and ate it up. Some fell on **rocky places**, where it did not have much soil. It sprang up quickly, because the soil was shallow. But when the sun came up, the plants were scorched, and they withered because they had no root. Other seed fell among **thorns**, which grew up and choked the plants. Still other seed fell on **good soil**, where it produced a crop—a hundred, sixty or thirty times what was sown."
—Matthew 13:3-8

Conversion is a process. ... Few of us make it in one big decision. Instead, it is a multitude of small choices—mini-decisions that a person makes toward Christ.[3]

—Jim Petersen

SPIRITUAL THERAPY

The process of helping patients overcome barriers and inviting them to take micro-steps of faith toward a healthy relationship with God.

37

Citations

1. Arn, W, Arn, C. *The Master's Plan for Making Disciples*. Baker Books, 1998.
2. Peterson, J. *Living Proof: Sharing the Gospel Naturally*. NavPress, 1988.

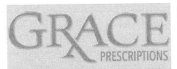

Understanding the Process of Spiritual Care

Key Questions

1. What are the phases of spiritual influence?
2. How do we diagnose and treat spiritual barriers?

The health professional/patient relationship presents significant opportunities for spiritual care. Understanding the fundamentals of spiritual influence will help you break through the barriers that arise on the patient's side, as well as on the health professional's side.

Case Study

Jennifer was excited about doing a rotation with Dr. Stewart, a well-known Christian physician, and was looking forward to seeing "faith in action." On her rotation, she was to take a history, including a spiritual history, do a brief exam, and arrive at a tentative diagnosis before meeting with her preceptor.

Whenever Dr. Stewart learned that the spiritual history indicated that the patient was not a Christian, his eyebrows would raise up and he would say, "Fresh meat! Let's march!"

After introducing himself, he would ask a few medical questions and then immediately launch into what he called eternal diagnosis questions such as, "I understand that you have never asked Jesus to come into your heart. Is that true?" Or, he might say, "I guess you know that we are all going to die someday. Do you feel you are ready to meet your maker?"

Then, he would pull a gospel tract out of his lab pocket and quickly share the tract. Jennifer never saw anyone pray the prayer, but Dr. Stewart assured her that many patients had prayed to receive Christ.

> Evangelism that ignores the wooing and tries to force a union misses the very heart of the new life in and with Jesus Christ. ... Give the bridegroom plenty of time to do His courting.[1]
>
> —Judy Gomboll

> For 15 years I said: "[We] are a harvest-oriented denomination living in the midst of an unseeded generation." We reduced planting, neglected cultivation, and not surprisingly have found the harvest coming up short. I now realize something more is going on. We are more like gardeners working the window boxes than farmers working the fields. We are the grandchildren of farmers keeping harvest stories alive over coffee and dessert at family reunions.[2]
>
> —Chuck Kelley

What do you admire about Dr. Stewart?

What is Dr. Stewart missing?

CULTIVATION: from Cynicism to Curiosity

History: _____ or _____

Diagnosis: The _____ barrier - a set of negative feelings toward Christianity that a person has allowed to develop, based on bad experiences with Christians or religious groups.

A reaction to bad _____

Prognosis: Individuals suffering from indifference and antagonism will suffer from isolation. As they withdraw, there will be no one to confront their mindset.

Approach: Build a bridge of caring relationship

Rx: Connection, faith flags, and acts of caring

Goal: _____, _____, and _____

PLANTING: from Curiosity to Understanding

History: _____

Diagnosis: The _____ barrier - a predisposition to disregard or reject Christianity

A reaction to bad _____

Prognosis: Individuals suffering from ignorance and error will move into indifference and perhaps hostility.

Approach: Presenting biblical truth that challenges the mind to consider Christ

Rx: Storytelling, apologetics, explanation, and clarification

Goal: _____ and _____

Angry Andrew: "Can you believe these Christians! They are so arrogant. How do they get off believing that they are so good that they are the only ones who get to go to heaven? Jerks!"

Sally Skeptic: "Dr. King, you're a really great doctor, but I'm just not interested in talking about religious stuff. I understand that this is really important to you and I respect that. But I'm just not interested."

Curious Chris: "This is all pretty interesting, but I've got a lot of questions. I'm just not ready to place my trust in a book thousands of years old. Besides, there are things I just can't swallow like the subjugation of women and the issue of slavery."

The antidote to isolation and ignorance is your presence and wise conversation as you build a bridge of caring relationship.

Doubting Thomas: "My life is good. If I became a Christian ... well, there are things I just don't want to give up."

As for you, you were dead in your transgressions and sins, in which you used to live when you followed the ways of this world and of the ruler of the kingdom of the air, the spirit who is now at work in those who are disobedient. All of us also lived among them at one time, gratifying the cravings of our sinful nature and following its desires and thoughts. Like the rest, we were by nature objects of wrath.
— Ephesians 2:1-3

Linda Legalist: "I can't stand spending time with my old friends. It's such a waste. I find myself preaching at them. It just makes everyone angry."

Cami Chameleon: "I love to go to church, but when I'm with my old friends, I want to please my friends more than I want to please God."

HARVEST: from Understanding to Trust

History: _____

Diagnosis: The _____ barrier - a predisposition to resist examining spiritual issues or to reject Christ outright based on a sinful nature.

A reaction to a bad _____

Prognosis: Indecision and love of the darkness result in pride and independence, which unchecked will be irreversible.

Approach: Meaningful discussion that continues to erode barriers, persuasion that speaks to the will, and prayer that cries to God for this person's conversion.

Rx: Continued conversation and prayer

Goal: _____

MULTIPLYING: from Trust to Reproduction

History: _____

Diagnosis: The _____ barrier – failure to balance truth and grace resulting in over-separation or over-identification

A reaction to a fallen _____

Prognosis: Unless spiritual infants find a home where they can be nurtured in truth *and* grace, their growth will be stunted and spiritual influence lost.

Approach: Integration into the body of Christ and discipleship

Rx: Opportunities to learn, serve, and worship

Goal: _____ and _____

41

> For the law was given through Moses; grace and truth came through Jesus Christ.
>
> —John 1:17

Balancing Truth and Grace[3]

OVER-SEPARATION	OVER-IDENTIFICATION
All about _____	All about _____
Holy Huddle	Acceptance
Legalism	Assimilation
Critical	Camouflaged
Radical Message	Radical Connection
No Audience	No Message
Porcupine	Chameleon
Lost Influence	Lost Influence

On Your Own

Identify five people (family, friend, or patient) you would like to see come to faith. What is the next barrier they need to overcome?

Name	Barrier
1. _____	_____
2. _____	_____
3. _____	_____
4. _____	_____
5. _____	_____

Citations

1. Gomboll, J. "Matchmaker, Matchmaker: What would happen if you began to see evangelism as introducing someone to the Savior—rather than as salesmanship?" *Discipleship Journal*. 1990(May/Jun);57:28. http://www.navpress.com/magazines/archives/article.aspx?id=13275
2. Kelley, C: Southern Baptist are the New Methodist, Lecture at New Orleans Baptist Theological Seminary, March 2009, http://www.nobts.edu/publications/News/NewMethodists3-09.html
3. Adapted from: Hinckley, KC. *Living Proof: A Small Group Discussion Guide*. CBMC/NavPress, 1990.

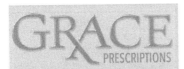

Module 8
Earning the Right to Be Heard

Key Questions

1. What are the foundational elements of building spiritual influence?
2. What are the characteristics of wise communication?

Be wise in the way you act toward outsiders; make the most of every opportunity. Let your conversation be always full of grace, seasoned with salt, so that you may know how to answer everyone.
—Colossians 4:5-6

Whatever you do, work at it with all your heart, as working for the Lord.
—Colossians 3:23

... in every way they will make the teaching about God our Savior attractive.
—Titus 2:10

Just like a great song, spiritual conversation needs both the right words as well as beautiful music. Without music, words can seem harsh and abrupt. Without lyrics, listeners are left too much on their own to determine the meaning of it all. Together, words and music have a deeper impact. The same is true of spiritual conversation. When the beauty of the message (lyrics) is supported by the beauty of your life (music), your patients will be attracted to your song.

Case Study

Jan is a 32-year-old single white female who has been your patient for three years. She works at a high-stress job and it's taken its toll on her physically. She's in to see you about worsening dental pain.

As you describe a possible procedure, Jane becomes more anxious and says that her roommate is trying to get her to see a spiritualist who uses herbs and spiritual "stuff." You marvel at her willingness to try something like this when she hasn't responded positively to spiritual conversation in the past.

You decide to take a chance and relate a brief story of how you found peace when you were faced with an illness. You conclude, "Jan, God didn't heal me immediately like I asked, but I found something more valuable. Through that experience, I developed a relationship with a God who walks through every problem with me. I'd love to tell you more sometime, if you're interested."

Jan's eyes tear up and she responds, "Maybe I need to know a God like that."

What would you do or say next?

How do you think she would respond if you . . .

- ▶ invited her to church?
- ▶ told her your testimony?
- ▶ told her how dangerous a spiritualist can be?
- ▶ pulled out a tract and went over it with her?
- ▶ gave her a faith prescription to memorize a verse?

The Foundation for Communication

Building a foundation for spiritual conversation is critical for spiritual therapy and involves four elements.

4.		
1.	**2.**	**3.**
▶ People don't care if you are a good person until they know that you do good work. ▶ If you want people to pay attention to your faith, you must first pay attention to your work.	▶ It's not enough to do good work. ▶ There must be something attractive about you personally.	▶ People don't care how much you know until they know how much you care. ▶ You show concern and compassion by what you say and do.

Five Principles of Wise Communication

1. **Are your words** _____?

    ▶   Why is it important to watch the spiritual jargon?

    ▶   What are some terms that might be confusing or might put off individuals who are not persons of faith?

2. **Are your words** _____ **and helpful?**

    ▶   Ecclesiastes 12:9-10

    ▶   Ephesians 4:29

3. **Does it include more than** _____?

Elements of Communication[2]

- ▸ Words alone _____
- ▸ Tone of voice _____
- ▸ Gesture/body language _____

4. **Is the person** _____ **in what you have to say?**

- ▸ 1 Peter 3:15

- ▸ Other interest indicators

5. **Are you more interested in the** _____
   with whom you are speaking or what you have to say?

- ▸ Focused listening

- ▸ Appropriate Touch

Important Principles

1. _____ interaction with every person is spiritually significant.

2. Spiritual influence is more about what _____ is doing than about what you do.

3. It's not about closing the deal; it's about being _____ link in a chain.

4. Our job is to find out what the _____ is doing and join Him.

5. What you _____ is more important than what you say—at first.

38%

55%

7%

Personal Exercise

Are you so compromised by the business of healthcare that you can't even consider these questions?

▶ Who is watching you?

▶ Do your words build walls or tear down walls?

▶ What is one thing you can do to help someone take the next step toward Jesus?

Citations

1. Trueblood, E. *The Company of the Committed*. Harper, 1961.
2. Mehrabian, A. Communication without Words. *Psychology Today.* 1968(Sep):53-55.

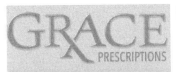

Module 9
Using Faith Flags, Faith Stories, and Faith Prescriptions

Key Questions
1. How can we identify a patient's interest and openness to discuss spiritual issues?
2. How can clinicians appropriately introduce faith discussions without offending a patient?

There are many ways to communicate truth, but a story has a unique power to grab our attention. They make truth come to life. It's why Jesus taught in parables and why we can use stories to awaken the hearts and intensify a hunger to know more about a relationship with God.

Case Study

David, a 35-year-old male, was referred to you for evaluation and treatment of suspected peptic ulcer disease. He readily shares with you that many things in his life are not going well. In addition to work stress, his marriage is on the rocks. On additional questioning, he confides that life has not turned out the way he had hoped.

It is clear that David realizes his disease is probably related to his life circumstances. He freely provides a spiritual history revealing that while he believes there is a God, he has not been connected with a religious community since he was a child.

You explain that our wellbeing requires that we be healthy physically, emotionally, and spiritually, and then you add that when you went through difficult time, it was your faith in God that pulled you through. David's response is, "Really?"

What would you do next?

Examples of Religious Jargon and alternatives:

Rather than:	Use:
Sin	Wrongdoing
Lost	Without a relationship with God
Salvation	Knowing God personally
Faith	Trust in
Repent	Change mind/heart

What can simple statements like this do in the lives of your patients?

How can you use faith flags in your practice?

What faith flags do you already use?

Raising Faith Flags

Definition

A casual comment in the course of a natural conversation in which you identify yourself as someone to whom God, faith, the Bible, or prayer is important.

Protocol

Faith flags …

- Are a _____ part of conversation
- Are _____
- Reveal that you have a _____ dimension
- Watch for (but do not demand) a _____
- Create _____ for further discussion

Faith flags avoid …

- Information _____
- Religious _____
- Identification with a church or _____
- Using faith as an _____ for doing or not doing something

Examples

In a conversation about a problem with a patient's children:

Some of our best ideas for raising our children came from the Bible.

Before or after a procedure:

Do you know anyone who could pray for you as you are recovering?

In a conversation about marital conflict:

I've been surprised to learn how much the Bible has to say about marriage.

During a discussion about depression:

I remember the time that I first heard what the Bible had to say about being discouraged.

Telling Faith Stories

Definition

A short account of how God, faith, prayer, a Bible verse, or a biblical principle has helped you, your family, your marriage, or one of your patients.

Protocol

Faith stories …

- ▶ Are a natural part of conversation

- ▶ Are short: one or _____ minutes maximum

- ▶ Focus on God, spiritual faith, prayer, or the Bible

- ▶ Correspond with a _____ in their life

- ▶ Provide a glimpse of the benefits of being God's _____

Faith stories avoid …

- ▶ Religious jargon

- ▶ Becoming a _____

- ▶ Identification with a church or denomination

- ▶ Pushing for a _____

- ▶ Attempts to _____

Examples

In a conversation where a mother expresses real concern about her child's pending medical procedure:

> *I'll never forget when my son was six and in the first grade, going through a day of tests at the hospital to see why he was experiencing petit mal seizures in class. He was a brave little trooper until the needle came out at the end of the day with the dye for the CAT scan. He and I both lost it at that point. I'll never forget how pain shrunk our world that day. Reality for me was limited to that 15x15 room. Pain can do that. It shrinks our world until there's no room even for God and we think we are all alone. But just because I couldn't sense or see Him didn't mean He wasn't there.*

In a conversation where a patient confesses being stressed over a difficult decision she had to make at work:

> It may surprise you to learn that many of the decisions I make to manage my medical practice are based on the Bible. One day, a friend of mine sat me down and showed me a bunch of principles in the Bible that could help make a successful business. I was floored to find so much practical information in such an old book. If you'd like, sometime I'd be happy to tell you what I learned.

In a conversation where a patient explains how his illness is forcing him to make a major change of plans:

> I still remember feeling just as disappointed as you seem to feel when my doctor told me I couldn't go on a long-awaited trip because of my sickness. At first, I got mad at God and said, "Lord, why are You doing this to me?" But after a few hours my attitude began to change, and I began to ask Him, "Lord, what are You doing?" During that recovery, I spent some time talking to God and reading His Word, and He used that time I had alone with Him to show me some things I could have learned no other way.

Faith Story Exercise

Step One: List some of the most frequent topics of conversation you've had with patients when you have sensed some kind of spiritual openness.

Step One: Frequent topics of conversation

Step Two: List spiritual experiences you have had that correspond with the list of topics you made in Step One.

Step Two: Corresponding personal spiritual experiences

Step Three: Choose one or two of these experiences and write a brief faith flag or story about each one.

Step Three: Your faith story

Faith Prescriptions

Definition

A recommendation to do, read, and/or watch something to help your patient, colleague, or friend take the next step in their spiritual journey.

Protocol

Faith prescriptions can be …

- ▶ Simple, verbal communication
- ▶ Written on script

Examples

To do:

- ▶ Memorize a verse or section of Scripture
- ▶ Begin a gratitude journal
- ▶ Pray or have a daily quiet time
- ▶ Talk to a pastor or a Christian counselor
- ▶ Take your spouse or child on a date
- ▶ Take your spouse or family on a trip
- ▶ Volunteer at a local ministry

To read:

- ▶ Read a portion of the Bible
- ▶ Read an article or chapter in a particular book
- ▶ Read material on a trusted internet site
- ▶ Purchase and read an item from Prescribe-a-Resource®

To watch:

- ▶ A particular video or video series
- ▶ A movie or documentary
- ▶ A special on TV

Download the CMDA Prescribe-a-Resource® App for free in the Apple App Store or visit *www.cmda.org/par*.[1]

Record the prescription in your medical record. When patients return for their next visit, check their compliance.

Summary

Faith flags, stories, and prescriptions are powerful ways of communicating spiritual truth to your patients.

They allow you to talk about God, spiritual faith, the Bible, and/or prayer without being pushy or intrusive, and can help patients consider whether they want to talk more about their spiritual needs.

Citations

1.   Prescribe-a-Resource® App. CMDA. 2013. *www.cmda.org/par*.

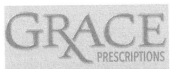

Your Personal Faith Story

One of the most important means of imparting spiritual insight to a patient is to describe your own spiritual journey in a brief personal faith story. It not only clarifies the elements of the Good News but also helps a person consider the conceivability of taking a step of faith themselves.

Case Study

Walt was raised in a nominally Christian home. Church was familiar, but having a personal relationship with Christ was not. While at the university, the gospel registered to him for the first time. He knew that there was something missing from his life. Here is his story.

After viewing the video of Walt's faith story, discuss in your group.

What was effective in the way this story was told?

Telling Your Story

One of the most effective ways to explain what it means to be a person of faith is to tell your personal faith story.

When telling your story ...

- ► Be sensitive to your listener

- ► Point out the specific needs or circumstances

- ► Limit details

- ► Focus on the good news

- ► Keep it positive

But in your hearts set apart Christ as Lord. Always be prepared to give an answer to everyone who asks you to give the reason for the hope that you have. But do this with gentleness and respect.
—1 Peter 3:15

When telling your story ...

- ▶ Avoid mentioning a specific _____

- ▶ Avoid _____

- ▶ Keep it _____

- ▶ Be personal, not _____

Get Organized

Paul's story in Acts 26 is a good outline.

- ▶ Opening: Acts 26:2-3
- ▶ Before: Acts 26:4-11
- ▶ How: Acts 26:12-20
- ▶ After: Acts 26:21-23
- ▶ Close: Acts 26:24-29

Group Exercise: Watch another video testimony then discuss in your groups:

- ▶ What was effective?
- ▶ What was ineffective?

Write Your Story

1. Using the next two pages, write out your personal faith story.

2. Describe the specific situation that led up to your salvation.

3. Describe how you trusted Christ.

4. Describe how Christ is currently affecting your life/meeting your needs.

5. Make a summary statement.

6. Ask for reflection.

If the world can write us off as super-spiritual people who don't have needs and problems like theirs, they'll write off God as irrelevant. But once they see and know that we are all alike, and that we have common needs and problems and interests, they'll be far more curious when we say, "God makes a difference."[1]

—Rebecca Pippert

As You Write
- ▶ Be authentic. Tell your story the way it happened.
- ▶ Identify one main idea or theme you want to communicate.
- ▶ Refrain from criticizing others.
- ▶ Read back through for jargon.

Your Faith Story

Describe the specific situation that led up to your salvation.

BEFORE

What were one or two of the deep inner longings that made you open to hearing about Christ?

How were you trying to solve these problems?

Were there any other circumstances that led you to feel your need of Christ?

Describe how you trusted Christ.

HOW

What were the specific events that led up to your acceptance of Christ?

How did you hear the gospel?

Was there a specific verse or passage of Scripture that hit you?

Was there a new thought that finally dawned upon you?

What were the specific steps you took to receive Christ?

AFTER
What is Christ doing in your life today?

How is Christ meeting your needs today?

Describe how Christ currently affects your life and is meeting your needs.

CLOSE
What summary statement can you make?
"My life isn't perfect, but I know that I have a relationship with Christ, and He
. . . can handle anything that comes my way."
. . . loves me unconditionally."
. . . says that I am valuable stuff."
. . . has given me a relationship with Him."
. . . says that I am forgiven."

Make a summary statement.

REFLECTION
"Has anything like this ever happened to you?"
"Has anyone ever taken the time to show you how the Bible says you can have a personal relationship with God?"
"May I share an illustration that explains how a person can receive forgiveness?"
"If this intrigues you, I would be glad to discuss this more sometime."

Ask for reflection.

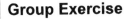

Group Exercise

In groups of two (three if necessary), share your faith stories and then discuss what elements of the stories are effective/ineffective.

Summary

The more you tell your story, the more natural it will become to you. Don't worry about memorizing it word for word. Just get down the key points you want to communicate and then watch for opportunities to tell your story.

Citations

1. Pippert, RC. *Out of the Saltshaker & Into the World: Evangelism as a Way of Life*. IVP Books, 1999.

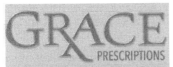

Module 11
Dealing with the Reality of Time

Inviting friends, colleagues, and patients to take a step toward God does not necessarily mean adding additional projects or tasks to an already impossible schedule. For most of us, it is a matter of being intentional in the routines of our lives and developing a team of gifted individuals to work with us—because we cannot do it alone.

Key Questions
1. When is it appropriate to talk more seriously about spiritual topics?
2. What are the basics of the Good News?
3. Given the time constraints of a busy practice, how can I communicate the Good News briefly?

Case Study

Jim Brennan is a cantankerous older patient who has continually ignored or resisted anything religious and lets you know about it. Over the last ten years, Dr. Richards has raised countless faith flags and explained the health benefits of faith—seemingly to no avail.

Then, on the morning of his appointment to hear his biopsy report, something changed. It was the peak of flu season and Dr. Richards was running behind. When he walked into Mr. Brennan's exam room over an hour late, instead of a verbal beating, he sensed that his patient's heart had softened.

"What's the word, Doc?" Mr. Brennan asked quietly.

Richards sighed and replied, "Jim, I've got bad news. It's cancer."

Mr. Brennan stared at the floor and said the unexpected: "Doc, I think I'm going to need that God you've been trying to tell me about for this one."

Have you ever encountered similar situations?

What is your assessment of the openness of these patients to discuss spiritual topics?

How would you respond to each patient?

Guidelines for Appropriate Spiritual Conversations

Recognizing an Open Door

Definition: An open door is an opportunity to talk more seriously about spiritual subjects at the invitation of the listener.

Identifying Doorknobs

Listen for ...

▶ Areas of _____

▶ Felt _____

▶ Previous _____ experience (positive or negative)

▶ Direct _____

Opening the Door

When broaching spiritual issues ...

▶ Proceed _____

▶ Ask _____

▶ Regulate the _____

Preparing for the Spiritual Emergency

If you consistently raise faith flags and tell faith stories, eventually you will be caught in a time crunch by someone who wants to know more. If you take time to talk with the person, you will back up the waiting room. But if you fail to take time, are you being unfaithful to God? How can you prepare to meet spiritual needs when they arise—even when it's inconvenient?

1. Develop a spiritual emergency _____.

2. Develop a spiritual _____ network.

3. Prepare _____.

Principles to Remember

Every opportunity is not an emergency.

I am not called to meet every need.

Saying "Yes" to someone always means saying no to someone else.

God has called others to meet needs besides me.

Two are better than one, because they have a good return for their labor: If either of them falls down, one can help the other up. But pity anyone who falls and has no one to help them up. Also, if two lie down together, they will keep warm. But how can one keep warm alone? Though one may be overpowered, two can defend themselves. A cord of three strands is not quickly broken.
—Ecclesiastes 4:9-12 (NIV 2011)

Four Questions to Ask in a "Spiritual Emergency"

1. Is it an emergency?

2. Am I the best one to handle this?

3. How will my decision affect others?

4. Is this the best time?

Building Your Spiritual Consult Team

▶ Evaluate your patients' _____.

▶ Determine what kinds of spiritual _____ are needed.

▶ Evaluate _____ skills, abilities, resources, and time, and determine the best part for you to play.

▶ Determine the kind of _____ you need (given your gifts).

▶ Consider the people in close _____: colleagues, staff, patients, chaplains.

▶ List _____ who have the skills and experience to help: pastors, friends, counselors.

▶ _____.

▶ Enlist their _____.

▶ Set up an emergency _____.

63

Identifying Your Potential Team

Make a list of your potential team members and the roles they can play and needs they can meet.

Name	Role/Need
_____	_____
_____	_____
_____	_____
_____	_____
_____	_____
_____	_____
_____	_____
_____	_____
_____	_____
_____	_____
_____	_____
_____	_____
_____	_____
_____	_____
_____	_____
_____	_____
_____	_____
_____	_____
_____	_____

Consider four issues:
1. Competence
2. Confidentiality
3. Culpability
4. Compassion

NOTE: A more detailed module on "Dealing with the Reality of Time" is available in the *Saline Solution* DVD available from CMDA.

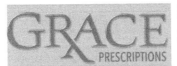

Module 12
Sharing the Good News

Key Questions
1. Given a patient's openness, how do I tell the Good News?
2. What is the best approach?

When it comes to sharing the Good News—whether with patients, staff, colleagues, or friends—a well thought-out plan and some preparation on your part will keep you focused on your patients' spiritual needs as you invite them to take the next step of faith.

Case Study

Dr. Scott Stringfield explains the Good News to patients by drawing a simple bridge diagram on exam table paper.

What did you like?

What are your patients' felt needs that the gospel addresses?

Telling the Good News

What's the Right Approach?

1. Does it answer the right core question?

   Every gospel presentation offers Jesus as the _____ to a personal felt need or aspiration.

   I need to know what an individual is _____ about and how the Good News addresses that concern.

"Unless they find a presentation of Christ surprisingly attractive and compelling (and stereotype breaking) their eyes will simply glaze over when you try to talk to them."[1]

—Tim Keller

2. Does it take into consideration the cultural assumptions that make Christianity seem implausible?

   Christianity can't be true because ...

   Our job is not necessarily to _____ cultural assumptions but cause doubt in their truth.

Consider: What might be so attractive about Christ and the gospel to your patient that would make them stop and listen?

3. Am I personally comfortable with it?

Telling the Good News (cont.)

One-verse Good News

> For the wages of sin is death, but the gift of God is eternal life in Christ Jesus our Lord.
>
> —Romans 6:23

Evaluation

▶ What did you like?

▶ What are the assumptions of this approach?

▶ What are the benefits/limitations?

▶ What is the best-fit scenario for this approach?

> People don't come to believe that they are sinners by being told. They have to be shown. People don't come to believe that they are loved by God by being told. They have to be shown.[2]
>
> —Tim Keller

Group Exercise

Discuss the following in your group:

What core questions do your patients express to you?

What effective ways have you found to answer them?

> You are the light of the world. A city on a hill cannot be hidden. Neither do people light a lamp and put it under a bowl. Instead they put it on its stand, and it gives light to everyone in the house. In the same way, let your light shine before men, that they may see your good deeds and praise your Father in heaven.
>
> —Matthew 5:14-16

What effective ways have you found to communicate the Good News?

Practicum

Using a tool with which you are comfortable, practice sharing the Good News to someone at your table. Use the space below if you want to draw something.

Citations

1. Keller, TJ. "Deconstructing Defeater Beliefs." Available at
    http://www.cominneapolis.org/sites/default/files/Deconstructing_Defeater_Beliefs_Tim_Keller.pdf
2. Keller, TJ. *The Reason for God: Belief in an Age of Skepticism.* Dutton, 2008.

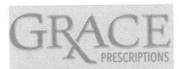

Praying with and for Patients

Prayer is one of the most potent tools in your armamentarium of patient care, not only because it has been shown by research to provide comfort for patients, but because ultimately God is the One who heals.

Key Questions

1. What is the place of personal and corporate prayer in a clinical practice?
2. How can clinicians appropriately pray with patients without offending them or violating ethical standards?
3. What are some potential pitfalls of praying with patients?
4. How will I integrate prayer into my practice?

Case Study

Susan's workup for chronic pain had failed to reveal a physical etiology. Though she initially resisted discussing her social and spiritual health, on re-questioning she was now willing to talk. She admitted that her marriage was on the rocks. And while she was active in her church, she did not know the peace that her pastor spoke about. Dr. Barbara asked Susan if she ever prayed about these things. She had not, but was willing to. As Dr. Barbara prayed, an emotional floodgate opened in Susan's heart.

Why Pray For or With Patients

What do you think? Discuss the following questions in your group:

 ▶ Do you think it is appropriate for health professionals to pray for or with their patients?

 ▶ Do you pray for or with your patients?

Four things let us ever keep in mind:
 ▶ God hears prayer,
 ▶ God heeds prayer,
 ▶ God answers prayer, and
 ▶ God delivers by prayer.[3]
　　　　　—E. M. Bounds

Encouragement Through the Ages

 ▶ "Pray as though everything depended on God. Work as though everything depended on you."[1]
　　　　　　　　　—Saint Augustine

 ▶ "As is the business of tailors to make clothes and cobblers to make shoes, so it is the business of Christians to pray."[2]
　　　　　　　　　—Martin Luther

 ▶ "Our prayer must not be self-centered. It must arise not only because we feel our own need as a burden we must lay upon God, but also because we are so bound up in love for our fellow men that we feel their need as acutely as our own. To make intercession for men is the most powerful and practical way in which we can express our love for them."[4]
　　　　　　　　　—John Calvin

The Biblical Case for Prayer

- The first time God calls on a man to pray it is for physical healing (Genesis 20:7).

- God prescribes prayer for Christians (1 Thessalonians 5:16-18).

- God prescribes prayer for the sick (James 5:14-15).

- God prescribes prayer for our time of need (Hebrews 4:16).

- God cares about the physical world and human bodies (Matthew 14:14; 3 John 1:2; 1 Thessalonians 5:23).

- God hears us (1 John 5:14-15).

- Ultimate healing comes from a relationship with Christ (Isaiah 53:4-5; Revelation 21:3-5).

The Clinical Case for Prayer

Patient Desire

Most patients draw on prayer and other religious resources to navigate and overcome the spiritual challenges that arise in their illnesses.[5]

- About _____ of physicians say patients sometimes or often mention spiritual issues such as prayer.[5]

- _____ of U.S. physicians believe the experience of illness often or always increases patients' awareness of and focus on religious/spiritual (R/S) issues.[5]

Patients desire prayer with their physician in certain instances.[6]

- Patient agreement with a health professional praying for them increases strongly with the _____ of the illness setting.[6]

- There is only 19% patient agreement with physician prayer in a routine office visit, but 29% agreement in a hospitalized setting, and 50% agreement in a life-threatening scenario.[6]

Physician Practice

Most physicians believe prayer is positive in healthcare.[5]

- Helps patients to cope (76%)

- Gives patients a positive state of mind (74%)

- Provides emotional and practical support via the religious community (55%)[5]

However, physicians are divided about when and if it is appropriate.[7] At least _____ of doctors sometimes engage in prayer with their patients.[7]

The Research

Several studies reported significant effects of intercessory prayer.

- ► Byrd RC, et al. *South Med J.* 1988;81:826–829.[23]
- ► Cha KY, et al. *J Reprod Med.* 2001;46(9):781–787.[24]
- ► Harris WS, et al. *Arch Intern Med.* 1999;159:2273–2278.[27]
  Lesniak KT. *Altern Ther Health Med.* 2006;12:42–48.[31]
- ► Matthews DA, et al. *South Med J.* 2000(Dec);93(12):1177–1186.[35]
- ► Sicher F, et al. *West J Med.* 1998;169(6):356–363.[40]

Including a retrospective study done 10 years after diagnosis:

- ► Leibovici L. *BMJ.* 2001;323:1450–1451.[33]

Some studies have been negative.

- ► Aviles JM, et al. *Mayo Clin Proc.* 2001;76(12):1192–1198.[20]
- ► Astin JA, et al. *Altern Ther Health Med.* 2006;12:36–41.[19]
- ► Krucoff MW, et al.. *Lancet.* 2005;366(9481):211–217.[29]

Including the largest and most rigorous trial:

- ► Benson H, et al. *Am Heart J.* 2006;151(4):934–942.[21]

Why the mixed results?

1. Scientific study of prayer's efficacy in healing is problematic.
   "God may indeed exist and prayer may indeed heal; however, it appears that, for important theological and scientific reasons, randomized controlled studies cannot be applied to the study of the efficacy of prayer in healing." [1]

   "In fact, no form of scientific enquiry presently available can suitably address the subject."[10]

2. Studies do not meet certain RCT standards.
   "All of the published studies fail to meet RCT standards in several critical respects. Primarily, they fail to measure and control exposure to prayer from others."[12]

3. Two important questions remain unanswered.
   If research on intercessory prayer is positive, does it suggest to us ways and means by which we can manipulate God or make His behavior statistically predictable?[10]

   Why would any divine entity be willing to submit to experiments that attempt to validate His existence and constrain His responses?[10]

The aim of science is not to open a door to infinite wisdom but to set a limit to infinite error.[11]

—Galileo

Praying with Patients

Rationale[13]

Harold Koenig, MD, wrote, "First, many patients are R/S (religious/spiritual) and have spiritual needs related to medical or psychiatric illness.

- ▶ "Studies of medical and psychiatric patients and those with terminal illnesses report that the vast majority have such needs, and most of those needs currently go unmet.

- ▶ "Unmet spiritual needs … can adversely affect health.

"Second, R/S influences the patient's ability to cope with illness.

- ▶ "In some areas of the country, 90% of hospitalized patients use religion (especially prayer) to enable them to cope with their illnesses and more than 40% indicate it is their primary coping behavior.

- ▶ "Poor coping has adverse effects on medical outcomes, both in terms of lengthening hospital stay and increasing mortality."[13]

Caution

Koenig advised:

"… contemplating a spiritual intervention (supporting R/S beliefs, praying with patients) should always be patient centered and patient desired. The health professional should never do anything related to R/S that involves coercion. The patient must feel in control and free to reveal or not reveal information about their spiritual lives or to engage or not engage in spiritual practices (i.e., prayer, etc.).

"In most cases, health professionals should not ask patients if they would like to pray with them, but rather leave the initiative to the patient to request prayer. The health professional, however, may inform R/S patients (based on the spiritual history) that they are open to praying with patients if that is what the patient wants.

"The patient is then free to initiate a request for prayer at a later time or future visit, should they desire prayer with the health professional."[13]

In our experience …
Most CMDA members are comfortable praying with and for patients, in at least some clinical situations.

Furthermore, after going through a CMDA training course (*Saline Solution* or *Grace Prescriptions*), Christian doctors seem even more willing and able to pray with and for patients in clinical practice.
—Larimore and Peel

If you choose to pray with patients, certain conditions should be considered beforehand.

Asking a patient if you can pray for them about a specific need can serve as a faith flag or a faith story.

If these conditions are not met, prayer led by the health professional has the potential to be coercive or harmful.

Prerequisites to Consider

1. Has a _____ history been taken?

2. Has the patient requested or _____ to prayer?

3. Do you and your patient hold _____ beliefs?

4. Does the _____ call for prayer?

Opportunities for Prayer

▶ Critical care

▶ Critical counseling

▶ Critical diagnosis

▶ Return of test results

▶ Hospice referral

▶ Preventive care visit

▶ Prenatal visit or birth of a baby

▶ Preoperative visit

▶ Other

Important Conditions

▶ Your patient's _____
  Does your patient even want you to pray with or for them? Or, not? Have you asked?

▶ Your patient's _____
  Will your patient give you permission to pray with or for them? Or, not? Have you asked?

▶ Your goal
  Is your goal to pray with each patient or is your goal to _____ each patient where they are in their spiritual journey?

Discuss with the patient

► Specific prayer _____, if any.

► Specific _____ with whom you can share the prayer request, if any (i.e., your nurse, your staff, prayer ministers at your church, etc.).

Praying Personally for Patients

The Priority

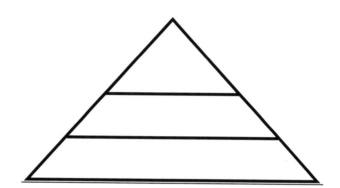

The Obligation

"Therefore confess your sins to each other and pray for each other so that you may be healed. The prayer of a righteous person is powerful and effective."

—James 5:16, NIV 2011

"Whether patients know it or not, want it or not, for Christian health professionals not to pray for and with their patients is as much spiritual malpractice as for pastors to fail to pray for their flock. For a patient who desires prayer, a Christian health professional's prayer for and with them may be as therapeutic as any other intervention he or she can offer."

—Walt Larimore, MD

"Not to employ prayer with my patients was the equivalent of deliberately withholding a potent drug or surgical procedure."[16]

—Larry Dossey, MD

Guidelines

Keep these things in mind if you are praying or requesting prayer for a patient without consent:

► If you ask others to pray, be 100% confident the patient cannot be identified.

► If you do reveal that fact to the patient ... be wise about when and how you reveal it.

Opportunities

Consider praying for your patients:

► During your daily quiet time

► While driving to and from work

► With other believers during the week or at worship times

► With other Christians at work (remembering HIPAA guidelines)

► Via an electronic prayer memo (remembering HIPAA guidelines)

Consider praying with your patients and/or their families:

► At the end of a patient encounter

► Before and/or after a procedure

► About a difficult clinical decision

Health Professionals' Quatrain[18]

► The grace of God

► The power of prayer

► The support of family and friends

► The miracle of modern medicine

Group Exercise

Discuss how prayer has been used as part of your practice. Discuss how you would like to incorporate it in the future.

Summary

As a Christian health professional, you have a powerful, healing resource not all health professionals know how to use—prayer. Use it! Wisely!

Addendum

Praying for Ourselves and our Patients

What We Can Pray for Ourselves

- That we would do excellent work (Proverbs 22:29)

- That we would bring glory to God (Matthew 5:16)

- We would treat people fairly (Colossians 4:1)

- We would have a good reputation with unbelievers (1 Thessalonians 4:12)

- Others would see Jesus in us (Philippians 2:12–16)

- Our lives would make our faith attractive (Titus 2:10)

- Our conversations would be wise, sensitive, grace-filled, and enticing (Colossians 4:5–6)

- We would be bold and fearless (Ephesians 6:19)

- We would be alert to open doors (Colossians 4:3)

- We would be able to clearly explain the gospel (Colossians 4:4)

- God would expand our influence (1 Chronicles 4:10)

What We Can Pray for Others[43]

- The Father would draw them to Himself (John 6:44)

- They would seek to know God (Deuteronomy 4:29; Acts 17:27) and would believe the Bible (Romans 10:17; 1 Thessalonians 2:13)

- Satan would be restrained from blinding them to the truth (Matthew 13:19; 2 Corinthians 4:4)

- The Holy Spirit would convict them of sin, righteousness, and judgment (John 16:8–13)

- God would send other Christians into their lives to influence them toward Jesus (Matthew 9:37–38)

- They would believe in Jesus as their Savior (John 1:12; 5:24)

- They would turn from sin (Acts 3:19; 17:30–31) and would confess Jesus as Lord (Romans 10:9–10)

- They would yield their lives to follow Jesus (Mark 8:34–37; Romans 12:1–2; 2 Corinthians 5:15; Philippians 3:7–8)

- They would take root and grow in Jesus (Colossians 2:6–7)

- They would become a positive influence for Jesus in their realm (2 Timothy 2:2)

Citations

1. BrainyQuote. http://www.brainyquote.com/quotes/quotes/s/saintaugus165165.html. This quote is also attributed to Ignatius of Loyola and D. L. Moody.
2. Christian Prayer Quotes. http://www.christian-prayer-quotes.christian-attorney.net.
3. Ibid.
4. Ibid.
5. Curlin, FA, Sellergren, SA, Lantos, JD, et al. Physicians' Observations and Interpretations of the Influence of Religion and Spirituality on Health. *Archives of Internal Medicine*. 2007(Apr);167(7):649-654.
6. MacLean, CD, Susi, B, Phifer, N, et al. Patient Preference for Physician Discussion and Practice of Spirituality. *Journal of General Internal Medicine*. 2003(Jan);18(1):38–43.
7. Monroe, MH, Bynum, D, Susi, B, et al. Primary care physician preferences regarding spiritual behavior in medical practice. *Archives of Internal Medicine*. 2003(Dec);163(22):2751-2756.
8. Peel, WC, Larimore, W. *Workplace Grace: Becoming a Spiritual Influence at Work*. Zondervan, 2010.
9. Berlinger, N. Quoted in: O'Reilly, KB. When a patient visit includes a request for prayer. *AMA News*. June 11, 2012.
10. Andrade, C, Radhakrishnan, R. Prayer and healing: A medical and scientific perspective on randomized controlled trials. *Indian Journal of Psychiatry*. 2009(Oct-Dec);51(4):247–253.
11. Galileo, Galilei. Quoted in: Brecht, B. *Life of Galileo*. Penguin Classics, 2008.
12. Sloan, RP, Ramakrishnan, R. Science, Medicine, and Intercessory Prayer. *Perspectives in Biology and Medicine*. 2006(Autumn);49(4):504–514.
13. Koenig, HG. Religion, Spirituality, and Health: The Research and Clinical Implications. *ISRN Psychiatry*. 2012, Article ID 278730.
14. BrainyQuote. http://www.brainyquote.com/quotes/quotes/m/martinluth385793.html.
15. Christian Prayer Quotes. http://www.christian-prayer-quotes.christian-attorney.net.
16. Dossey, L. *Healing Words: The Power of Prayer and the Practice of Medicine*. HarperOne, 1995.
17. Baxter, JS. Quoted in: Jones, C, Kelly, B. *The Tremendous Power of Prayer*. Howard Books, 2000.
18. Weir, A. "Quatrain." CMDA Weekly Devotion. January 8, 2013. http://www.cmda.org/WCM/CMDA/MinistryOutreaches2/Church_Resources1/WeeklyDevotions/Devotions1/Tuesday_January_8_2013_Quatrain.aspx.
19. Astin, JA, Stone, J, Abrams, DI, Moore, DH, et al. The efficacy of distant healing for human immunodeficiency virus-results of a randomized trial. *Alternative Therapies in Health and Medicine*. 2006;12:36–41.
20. Aviles, JM, Whelan, SE, Hernke, DA, et al. Intercessory prayer and cardiovascular disease progression in a coronary care unit population: A randomized controlled trial. *Mayo Clinic Proceedings*. 2001;76(12):1192–1198.
21. Benson, H, Dusek, JA, Sherwood, JB, et al. Study of the Therapeutic Effects of Intercessory Prayer (STEP) in cardiac bypass patients: A multicenter randomized trial of uncertainty and certainty of receiving intercessory prayer. *American Heart Journal*. 2006;151(4):934–942.
22. Burke, B. *Does God Still Do Miracles?* Victor, 2006.
23. Byrd, RC. Positive therapeutic effects of intercessory prayer in a coronary care unit population. *Southern Medical Journal*. 1988;81:826–829.
24. Cha, KY, Worth, DP. Does prayer influence the success of in vitro fertilization-embryo transfer? Report of a masked, randomized trial. *Journal of Reproductive Medicine*. 2001;46(9):781–787.
25. Curlin, FA, Chin, MH, Sellergren, SA, et al. The Association of Physicians' Religious Characteristics With Their Attitudes and Self-Reported Behaviors Regarding Religion and Spirituality in the Clinical Encounter. *Medical Care*. 2006(May);44(5):446-453.
26. Curlin, FA, Sellergren, SA, Lantos, JD, et al. Physicians' Observations and Interpretations of the Influence of Religion and Spirituality on Health. *Archives of Internal Medicine*. 2007(Apr);167(7):649-654.
27. Harris, WS, Gowda, M, Kolb, JW, et al. A randomized, controlled trial of the effects of remote, intercessory prayer on outcomes in patients admitted to the coronary care unit. *Archives of Internal Medicine*. 1999;159:2273–2278.
28. Koenig, HG. Religion, Spirituality, and Health: The Research and Clinical Implications. *ISRN Psychiatry*. 2012, Article ID 278730.
29. Krucoff, MW, Crater, SW, Gallup, D, et al. Music, imagery, touch, and prayer as adjuncts to interventional cardiac care: The Monitoring and Actualisation of Noetic Trainings (MANTRA) II randomised study. *Lancet*. 2005;366(9481):211–217.
30. Larimore, W, Peel, WC. *The Saline Solution: Sharing Christ in a Busy Practice*. Christian Medical & Dental Associations, 2000.
31. Lesniak, KT. The effect of intercessory prayer on wound healing in nonhuman primates. *Alternative Therapies in Health and Medicine*. 2006;12:42–48.
32. Levy, D, Kilpatrick, J. *Gray Matter: A Neurosurgeon Discovers the Power of Prayer*. Tyndale House Publishers, 2011.
33. Leibovici, L. Effects of remote, retroactive intercessory prayer on outcomes in patients with bloodstream infection: In randomised controlled trial. *BMJ*. 2001;323:1450–1451.
34. MacLean, CD, Susi, B, Phifer, N, et al. Patient Preference for Physician Discussion and Practice of Spirituality. *Journal of General Internal Medicine*. 2003(Jan);18(1):38–43.

35. Matthews, DA, Marlowe, SM, MacNutt, FS. Effects of intercessory prayer on patients with rheumatoid arthritis. *Southern Medical Journal*. 2000(Dec);93(12):1177-1186.

36. Matthews, DA, Clark, C. *The Faith Factor: Proof of the Healing Power of Prayer*. Penguin Books, 1999.

37. Monroe, MH, Bynum, D, Susi, B, et al. Primary care physician preferences regarding spiritual behavior in medical practice. *Archives of Internal Medicine*. 2003(Dec);163(22):2751-2756.

38. O'Reilly, KB. When a patient visit includes a request for prayer. *AMA News*. June 11, 2012.

39. Peel, WC, Larimore, W. *Workplace Grace: Becoming a Spiritual Influence at Work*. Zondervan, 2010.

40. Sicher, F, Targ, E, Moore, D, et al. A randomized double blind study of the effect of distant healing in a population with advanced AIDS. Report of a small scale study. *Western Journal of Medicine*. 1998;169(6):356–363.

41. Sloan, RP, Ramakrishnan, R. Science, Medicine, and Intercessory Prayer. *Perspectives in Biology and Medicine*. 2006(Autumn);49(4):504–514.

42. Weir, A. "Quatrain." CMDA Weekly Devotion. January 8, 2013.

43. Adapted from: Hinckley, KC. *Living Proof: A Small Group Discussion Guide*. CBMC/NavPress, 1990.

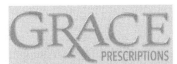

Module 14
Conclusion

Key Questions
1. What are four important imperatives for spiritual influence?
2. How can I specifically pray for myself and my patients?

You are the salt of the earth. But if the salt loses its saltiness, how can it be made salty again? It is no longer good for anything, except to be thrown out and trampled underfoot.
—Matthew 5:13 (NIV 2011)

Let your conversation be always full of grace, seasoned with salt.
—Colossians 4:6a

You are the light of the world. A town built on a hill cannot be hidden. Neither do people light a lamp and put it under a bowl. Instead they put it on its stand, and it gives light to everyone in the house.
—Matthew 5:14-15

Be wise in the way you act toward outsiders; make the most of every opportunity.
—Colossians 4:5

Spiritual care for patients is not only appropriate, it is a standard of care. Inviting friends, colleagues, and patients to take a step toward God is one of the greatest privileges and joys of being a child of God.

Final Thoughts

Becoming a person of spiritual influence demands at least four things.

1. **It takes** _____.
   - ▶ By consistently demonstrating competence in our work, godliness in our character, and compassion in our words and deeds.
   - ▶ Gracious words create a thirst to know more.

2. **It takes** _____.
   - ▶ Intentionally engaging non-Christians in order to show them the love of Jesus.
   - ▶ Remembering every interaction with every person is spiritually significant.
   - ▶ Using faith stories to let someone see what it's like to be a child of God.
   - ▶ Becoming comfortable with a way to share God's story of Good News.
   - ▶ Relating your own personal faith story.
   - ▶ Planning ahead by developing a spiritual emergency protocol and assembling a spiritual referral network.

3. **It takes** _____.
   - ▶ Remembering evangelism is a process.
   - ▶ Taking a spiritual history to assess spiritual needs and readiness.
   - ▶ Raising faith flags and watching for open doors.
   - ▶ Stopping to ask "What is God Doing? (WIGD) before we speak.

> The prayer of a righteous person is powerful and effective.
>
> —James 5:16b

4. **It takes** _____.

▶ Remembering to pray for yourself.

▶ Remembering that spiritual influence is more about what God is doing than about what you do.

▶ Praying *for* patients always, and *with* patients when appropriate.

▶ Asking the Spirit about what He is doing and for permission to join Him.

Personal Application

Consider the following questions and record your thoughts:

What are the implications of this material for my current situation?

What are the implications of this material for my (future) practice?

How will I communicate these principles to my colleagues?

Which of the following ideas should I consider?

- ☐ Use the G-O-D spiritual history questions that naturally bring up prayer.
- ☐ Pray during rounds when you sense an openness and the Holy Spirit's leading.
- ☐ Pray during office visits when you sense the Holy Spirit's leading.
- ☐ Ask permission before you pray.
- ☐ Attempt to pray for every patient in some way.
- ☐ Enlist your staff to pray, considering HIPAA regulations.
- ☐ Ask patients to pray with or for you.
- ☐ Pray for staff and colleagues.
- ☐ Form a prayer network for caregivers, staff, and/or patients.
- ☐ Engage a pastor or healthcare chaplain to pray with patients.
- ☐ Set up a prayer room in your clinic.
- ☐ Work with your chaplains or local pastors to establish an intercessory prayer network.
- ☐ Establish a weekly prayer gathering for staff, patients, doctors, and patients.
- ☐ Other _____

_____

_____

_____

Recommended Resources

1. Arn, W, Arn C. *The Master's Plan for Making Disciples*. Baker Books, 1998.
2. Barna, G. *Evangelism that Works*. Regal Books, 1995.
3. Burke, B. *Does God Still Do Miracles?* Victor, 2006.
4. Koenig, H. *Spirituality in Patient Care: Why, How, When, and What*. Templeton Press, 2013.
5. Koenig, H, King, D, Carson, VB. *Handbook of Religion and Health – Second Edition*. Oxford University Press, 2012.
6. Larimore, W, Peel, WC. *The Saline Solution: Sharing Christ in a Busy Practice*. Christian Medical & Dental Associations, 2000.
7. Levy, D, Kilpatrick, J. *Gray Matter: A Neurosurgeon Discovers the Power of Prayer*. Tyndale House Publishers, 2011.
8. Martin, R. *Just Add Water – Christian Apologetics for Health Professionals*. Christian Medical & Dental Associations, 2005.
9. Matthews, DA, Clark, C. *The Faith Factor: Proof of the Healing Power of Prayer*. Penguin Books, 1999.
10. Peel, B. *What God Does When Men Lead*. Tyndale, 2009.
11. Peel, B, Larimore, W. *Workplace Grace: Becoming a Spiritual Influence at Work*. Zondervan Publishers, 2010.
12. Rudd, G, Weir, A. *Practice by the Book: A Doctor's Guide to Living and Serving*. Christian Medical & Dental Associations, 2005.
13. Sala, HJ, Tada, JE. *What You Need to Know About Healing: A Physical and Spiritual Guide*. B&H Books, 2013.
14. Simpson, ML. *Permission Evangelism: When to Talk, When to Walk*. Cook Communications, 2004.
15. Stevens, D. *Just Add Water – Marks of a Christian Doctor*. Christian Medical & Dental Associations, 2004.
16. Stevens, D, Jones, B. *Leadership Proverbs: Wisdom for Today's Leaders*. Christian Medical & Dental Associations, 2010.
17. Stevens, D, Lewis, G. *Jesus, M.D.* Zondervan, 2001.
18. Stevens, D, et al. *Evangelism: Bridges to Other Faiths (CD)*. Christian Medical & Dental Associations, 2004.

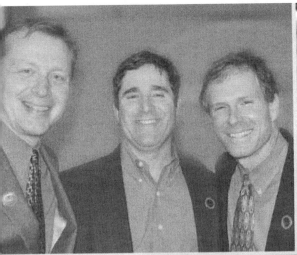
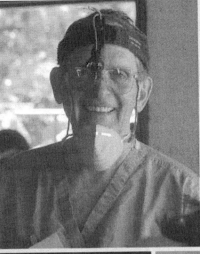
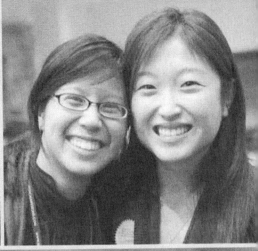
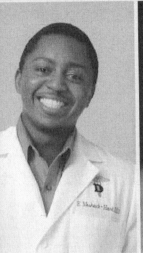
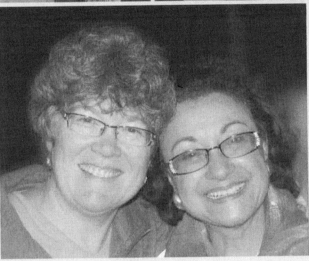
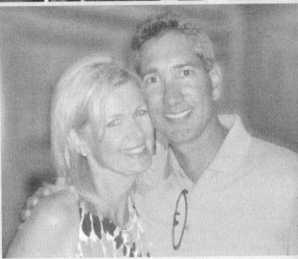

THE MANY FACES OF CMDA

PRACTICING PHYSICIANS AND DENTISTS	INTERNATIONAL AND DOMESTIC MISSIONARIES	RETIRED PHYSICIANS AND DENTISTS	UNIFORMED SERVICES
STUDENTS AND RESIDENTS	PRACTICING ASSOCIATES	SPOUSES AND FRIENDS	LIFETIME MEMBERS

JOIN US

Join the thousands of Christian healthcare professionals who seek
to change the face of healthcare by changing hearts in healthcare

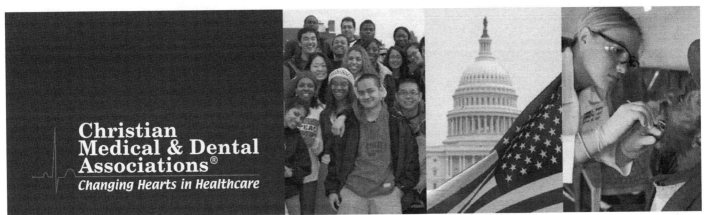

P.O. Box 7500 • Bristol, TN 37621 • 423-844-1000 • 888-230-2637 • *www.joincmda.org*

ECFA
Enhancing Trust

Membership Application

First Name   MI   Last Name   Degree

Home Address   Apt.

City   State   ZIP

Home Phone   Cell Phone

Permanent Email Address *Required*

Birth Date   Male/Female

Statement of Faith

While each of us holds fast to additional beliefs important to our relationship with God, the following statement outlines the tenets that provide a foundation for our fellowship and participation in the Christian Medical & Dental Associations.

I believe:
- In the divine inspiration and final authority of the Bible as the Word of God;
- In the eternal God revealed in Holy Scripture as Father, Son and Holy Spirit;
- In the unique Deity of Jesus Christ, God's only Son, whose death and resurrection provide by grace through faith the only means of my salvation;
- In the transforming presence and power of the Holy Spirit.

REQUIRED: Signature _____

Additional information on back

Membership Categories and Dues *Please check all that apply.*

Graduate Doctors
(MD, DDS, DMD, DO, DPM)
- ❏ With a practice
- ❏ Without a practice
- ❏ Academic

Dues: $358

- ❏ Uniformed Service
- ❏ Graduate doctor - first year in practice

Dues: $179

Residents, Special Graduate Doctors, Associates, Others
- ❏ Residents
  ___ First year ___ Second year ___ Third year
- ❏ Fellow
- ❏ Missionary
- ❏ Associate Health Professional (PA, NP)
- ❏ Allied Health Professional
- ❏ PhD
- ❏ Non-healthcare organization

Dues: $99

- ❏ Missionary electronic-only option (email content instead of print magazine, CD or other physical materials)

Dues: FREE

Retired
Partially retired (working 1-20 hours weekly) OR
Fully retired (working 0 hours weekly)
- ❏ Graduate - **$164** OR **$81**
- ❏ Uniformed Service - **$81** OR **$52**
- ❏ Missionary - **$52**
- ❏ Associate Health Professionals - **$52**

Non-Healthcare
- ❏ Non-healthcare professional

Dues: $55

- ❏ Lifetime Membership. You can save money and never receive a dues notice again. For lifetime dues rates, visit *www.joincmda.org*, email *join@cmda.org* or call 888-230-2637.

- ❏ Dues Grace. If you are unable to pay your dues in full, you may choose a full dues waiver or make a one-time payment for whatever portion of this year's dues you can afford. We will consider your dues paid in full for the year.

Student Membership Categories and Dues

Pre-Medical or Dental Student
Year in Program:
- ❏ 1st Year ❏ 2nd Year ❏ 3rd Year ❏ 4th Year

Medical or Dental Student
Year in Program:
- ❏ 1st Year ❏ 2nd Year ❏ 3rd Year ❏ 4th Year

Pending Degree _____

Associate Health or PhD Student
Year in Program:
- ❏ 1st Year ❏ 2nd Year ❏ 3rd Year ❏ 4th Year

Pending Degree _____

CMDA offers two types of student membership:
1. **Subscription:** This allows you to receive CMDA publications (including *Today's Christian Doctor* and *Christian Doctor's Digest*) in hard copy format.
   Dues: $55

2. **Electronic:** This allows you to receive publications and all other communications from CMDA via email and our website.
   Dues: FREE

Please circle your membership type here:

Subscription   OR   Electronic

Student / Resident Applicants:

_____

Name of School   City & State

_____

Expected Year of Completion   Program Length

Payment

Enclosed is my check for $ _____

Please charge my: ❏ Visa ❏ Mastercard ❏ American Express ❏ Discover $ _____

Card Number _____   Exp. Date _____

Signature of Card Holder _____   Phone (___) _____

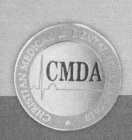
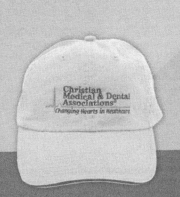
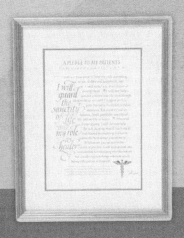
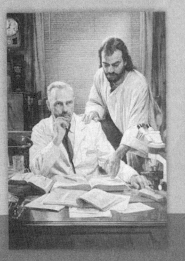

Grace Prescriptions Evaluation

Thank you for participating in the Grace Prescriptions Seminar! Please take a few minutes to answer the questions below so that we may continue to make the program better. You can complete this form and submit it by one of the methods listed below or complete it online at www.surveymonkey.com/s/gracerx. May the Lord richly bless you as you put into practice the principles learned through this seminar!

Seminar Location _____ **Date(s)**_____

Type of Seminar
- ☐ Live   Presenter(s): _____

- ☐ DVD Series   Moderator(s): _____

How did you learn of the conference? (Check all that apply)
    Advertisement: ☐ Today's Christian Doctor   ☐ Christian Doctor's Digest
    ☐ Email blast or electronic flyer
    ☐ Word of mouth / personal invitation: By whom? _____
    ☐ Social Media: Which form? _____
    ☐ Website: Which site? _____
    ☐ Other _____

What sessions did you find most helpful?

What sessions were not as helpful?

How will this course change your practice/life?

What suggestions do you have for improvements?

Indicate the appropriate rating using the following scale:
N/A=Not applicable   **1** = Poor   **2** = Fair   **3** = Average   **4** = Above Average   **5** = Outstanding

Quality of the content	N/A	1	2	3	4	5
Quality of the visual aids	N/A	1	2	3	4	5
Quality of the speakers	N/A	1	2	3	4	5
Usefulness to your practice and/or life	N/A	1	2	3	4	5
Registration procedure	N/A	1	2	3	4	5
Facility	N/A	1	2	3	4	5
Food quality & service	N/A	1	2	3	4	5
Overall conference organization	N/A	1	2	3	4	5

Additional comments? Please use the reverse side to make any additional comments you may have.

Submit form:
    Online: www.surveymonkey.com/gracerx   Mail: CMDA, P.O. Box 7500, Bristol, TN 37621
    Scan/Email: meetings@cmda.org   Fax: 423-844-1017